NCLEX® Review

Strategies and Skills

Nancy DiDona, EdD, RNC
Associate Professor of Nursing
Coordinator, Traditional Program of Nursing
Dominican College
Orangeburg, New York

D1455848

JONES AND BARTLETT PUBLISHERS
Sudbury, Massachusetts
BOSTON   TORONTO   LONDON   SINGAPORE

05/08

World Headquarters

Jones and Bartlett Publishers
40 Tall Pine Drive
Sudbury, MA 01776
978-443-5000
info@jbpub.com
www.jbpub.com

Jones and Bartlett Publishers
Canada
6339 Ormindale Way
Mississauga, Ontario L5V 1J2
Canada

Jones and Bartlett Publishers
International
Barb House, Barb Mews
London W6 7PA
United Kingdom

Jones and Bartlett's books and products are available through most bookstores and online booksellers. To contact Jones and Bartlett Publishers directly, call 800-832-0034, fax 978-443-8000, or visit our website www.jbpub.com.

Substantial discounts on bulk quantities of Jones and Bartlett's publications are available to corporations, professional associations, and other qualified organizations. For details and specific discount information, contact the special sales department at Jones and Bartlett via the above contact information or send an email to specialsales@jbpub.com.

The authors, editor, and publisher have made every effort to provide accurate information. However, they are not responsible for errors, omissions, or for any outcomes related to the use of the contents of this book and take no responsibility for the use of the products and procedures described. Treatments and side effects described in this book may not be applicable to all people; likewise, some people may require a dose or experience a side effect that is not described herein. Drugs and medical devices are discussed that may have limited availability controlled by the Food and Drug Administration (FDA) for use only in a research study or clinical trial. Research, clinical practice, and government regulations often change the accepted standard in this field. When consideration is being given to use of any drug in the clinical setting, the health care provider or reader is responsible for determining FDA status of the drug, reading the package insert, and reviewing prescribing information for the most up-to-date recommendations on dose, precautions, and contraindications, and determining the appropriate usage for the product. This is especially important in the case of drugs that are new or seldom used.

Library of Congress Cataloging-in-Publication Data
DiDona, Nancy A.
  NCLEX review : strategies and skills / Nancy DiDona.
    p. ; cm.
  Includes bibliographical references.
  ISBN-13: 978-0-7637-5226-2 (pbk. : alk. paper)
  ISBN-10: 0-7637-5226-6 (pbk. : alk. paper)
  1. Nursing--Examinations, questions, etc. 2. National Council Licensure Examination for Registered Nurses--Study guides. I. Title.
  [DNLM: 1. Nursing--Examination Questions. WY 18.2 D557n 2009]
  RT55.D53 2009
  610.73--dc22
                                    2008004912
6048

Production Credits
Executive Editor: Kevin Sullivan
Acquisitions Editor: Emily Ekle
Acquisitions Editor: Amy Sibley
Editorial Assistant: Patricia Donnelly
Production Director: Amy Rose
Production Editor: Carolyn F. Rogers
Associate Marketing Manager: Ilana Goddess
Manufacturing and Inventory Control Supervisor: Amy Bacus
Composition and Interior Design: Arlene Apone
Cover Design: Kristin E. Ohlin
Cover Image: © ErickN/ShutterStock, Inc.
Printing and Binding: Malloy, Inc.
Cover Printing: Malloy, Inc.

Printed in the United States of America
12 11 10 09 08 10 9 8 7 6 5 4 3 2 1

DEDICATION

I proudly dedicate this text to my husband Bob. During the recent year we became "empty-nesters" and celebrated our 33rd year of marriage. Bob has been my support, my confidant, and my morale booster. I love you and owe my success to your unending and unconditional love. Thank you.

I also dedicate this book to my wonderful sons, Robert and Gregory, and their loving and beautiful wives, Rebecca and Lori, and to all my amazing grandchildren. Many thanks for the encouraging words that have helped to sustain me in my work. Thank you.

To Gloria C. and Charles V.: You were there in the beginning, and I still feel your influence each time I teach the 5-Step Approach. Thank you.

CONTENTS

PREFACE

In 1990 two colleagues and I came together to develop a system that would assist our graduating students to pass the NCLEX®. We taught both licensed practical nursing students and registered professional nursing students. The NCLEX® passage rate at our school was acceptable and within the standards of the national average, but we believed this percentage could be improved. We developed a 5-Step Approach (see Chapter 4) and taught the process to a group of students. We sent the students to the board for testing and had a 92% passage rate. We decided to improve this percentage, and consequently we refined the process over the next year.

It was taught to a second group of students in 1991. This group of students achieved a 98% passage rate. In 1992 one of my colleagues passed away and the other went on to pursue a wonderful career. I took over teaching the 5-Step Approach shortly afterward, and I have refined and taught the process ever since.

It is wonderful to report that every student I determined to be ready to take the NCLEX® boards has passed. The skills and strategies I developed and the criteria to determine preparedness for testing are presented in this text. Read it, try it, and, most importantly, practice it! Repetition is the key that unlocks the powers of the 5-Step Approach.

Welcome to a new world of NCLEX® preparation! This text is designed to offer the reader a new and innovative way of preparing to successfully take the NCLEX-RN® and NCLEX-PN®. This is no "run-of-the-mill" NCLEX prepping text. There are many varieties of NCLEX preparation books on the market today, but none compares to the exciting and established techniques presented in this text. The most common types of NCLEX preparation texts being sold today include comprehensive review books and multiple question review books. These texts usually devote a few short pages at the beginning of the book for the purpose of explaining to the reader how to incorporate test-taking skills and strategies into answering the questions and describing the new NCLEX-RN and NCLEX-PN test plans. The brevity of this material seems to diminish the importance of the information. In reality, the introductory content is, or should be, rich with invaluable know-how and directions to accurately answering NCLEX questions. The remainder of the book is typically hundreds of questions, with or without content outline chapters.

A different approach is found in the pages of this text. What this text offers to the reader is a book that dedicates a significant amount of subject matter outlining skills and strategies useful in answering NCLEX style questions. Sufficient numbers of questions are also included for practice, and clearly defined outlines are provided that discuss knowing and understanding the NCLEX test plans. This is the kind of useful information that assists the test-taker in reaching the correct answer. The reason for this is simple. It is not possible for test-takers to know or remember all the content from all the healthcare subjects taught in nursing school. But test-takers are expected to critically think in choosing the right answer no matter how intricate the content area may be. How then is a test-taker supposed to do this? The answer can be explained two ways. First, the test-taker should begin a review having sufficient knowledge of the

> Review nursing content as needed.

NCLEX, NCLEX-RN, and NCLEX-PN are registered trademarks of the National Council of State Boards of Nursing, Inc.

nursing curriculum. If there is doubt in the test-taker's recall of nursing content, it is strongly suggested that a content review be completed concurrent with using this text. Second, the test-taker should use skills and strategies that assist him or her in arriving at the correct answer, even when the content area is unfamiliar or vague.

The concepts outlined in the pages to follow are fresh, original, and proven to be reliable and valid. The tactics learned from this text will assist a test-taker to be successful on most standardized examinations and are also beneficial to nursing students who are taking nursing courses and must pass school examinations designed analogous to the NCLEX test plan. Once a student becomes proficient in the skills and strategies discussed here, he or she is better able to apply them in a variety of learning situations.

As the uniqueness of this text unfolds, it becomes evident that the focus is on skills and strategies useful in answering NCLEX-type questions. The chapters include anecdotes from test-takers who have mastered these techniques, quips collected from years of trial and error in perfecting the methods presented, and invaluable hints, "tricks," and proven guidelines. When applicable, each chapter includes questions representative of the skill or strategy highlighted in the chapter, along with answers and rationales. Good luck!

WHAT IS A SKILL?

When a person is thought to possess a particular skill, it is generally believed he or she holds an ability or expertise that demonstrates proficiency in an area or a specific competence. A knack, if you will. This is what the test-taker will learn—the skills needed to answer NCLEX-style questions accurately. We have all heard others say they cannot take standardized tests or they are too nervous to pass standardized exams or they are not good when it comes to prepared tests. More often than not, the reason is test anxiety. And test anxiety comes from lack of preparation and defi-

> Knowing skills and strategies decreases test anxiety.

cient knowledge in testing practices. By this I mean not merely studying for a particular test or not learning the appropriate content. I mean not having sufficient skills or assistive maneuvers to help a person conclude the right answer. This is what you will acquire in the pages that follow. Skills are discussed that will guide you and help you to critically think. Your ability to read a question and deduce the correct answer will increase dramatically as you move toward becoming an authority in answering multiple choice questions and alternate format questions.

WHAT IS A STRATEGY?

When someone formulates a strategy, he or she devises a plan of action or designs an approach to achieve a goal. The goal here, naturally, is to pass the NCLEX. It therefore is necessary for you to learn the tactics and devices that can assist you in attaining your objective—becoming a licensed registered professional nurse or a licensed practical/vocational nurse. You will learn a new style in your approach to answering standardized test questions. This style incorporates the methodology necessary to sift through unnecessary information and target only what is relevant in selecting the right answer. It is not enough for a test-taker to feel satisfied with the level of understanding he or she attains in studying for a licensure examination. But if a test-taker combines this level of knowledge with tried and true test-taking strategies, success is inevitable.

Developing and Nurturing Skills and Strategies

Preparedness is the key to passing the NCLEX. Knowing the curriculum content, familiarizing oneself with the medications associated with different ailments, understanding standards of practice, and memorizing factual data are all important when facing any standardized test, but these are not enough. What is an important additional approach is the development and nurturing of test-taking skills and strategies. When developing these techniques, the ones that seem to have a comfortable "fit" should be chosen.

However, the ones that do not seem to have a comfortable fit should also be chosen, because the more uncomfortable a skill or strategy appears to be, the more change that will be associated with using the technique repeatedly. And changing your routine for answering standardized test questions is <u>essential</u> in increasing your proficiency in selecting the correct answer. Give yourself time to understand and practice the new concepts presented in this text. Then give yourself time to cultivate a mental connection for using the skills and strategies you have learned. This change will not occur rapidly. It may be subtle in its growth but it will take place! The idea is to change one pattern for another, to break down one habit to build another.

Habits: They Can Hurt You

It is a common belief that we are all creatures of habit. Some of our habits may be productive, and some may be destructive. Some habits do nothing but serve as comforting behaviors that help to control our stress and anxiety. What makes a behavior a habit is when the behavior occurs without conscience thought or premeditation. It is an involuntary action that happens automatically and makes us feel somewhat at ease with the turmoil or worry we are facing at the time.

As students, you have learned at an early age how to answer different types of questions on tests. Some were multiple choice, whereas others were fill in the blank, matching, and short answers. When you entered nursing school, you more than likely brought these test-taking habits with you and have used them throughout your nursing education. These behaviors obviously served you well, so why should you want to change them now? Because at one of the most stressful times in a test-takers life, and facing the NCLEX certainly falls into that category, you should be prepared to the best of your ability. That means being armed with the most current skills and strategies and being in the most primed state of mind and body. This is accomplished by replacing old test-taking habits with new habits. This is not easily done but is highly attainable.

First, you must deal with the resistance of your subconscious. With persistence, your involuntary state of mind that has dictated how you take a test will wave the proverbial flag of surrender and relinquish those old test-taking behaviors. How is this accomplished? Repetition, repetition, repetition! To replace any behavior with another, you must perform the new behavior repeatedly. If this is done, your subconscious mind *learns* to use the new behavior in place of the old. The new behavior in this case is applying the skills and strategies you learn from this text. But you must be diligent in practicing the new behaviors. This diligence allows your mind and body to *automatically* apply the behaviors to every question you answer on the NCLEX. Promise yourself that from this moment on you will only answer questions using the new behaviors you are about to learn. Make a commitment to changing your old habit and adopting a new and exciting habit for success on the NCLEX. I cannot stress the importance in making this commitment. It is vital to your success. The reason is that when confronted with stress or anxiety, we naturally turn to our habits to increase our comfort levels. When faced with the challenge of the NCLEX, if the new behaviors have not become your new test-taking habit, your mind will involuntarily return to the behaviors that support your old test-taking habit. From today on, answer practice questions using only the newly acquired skills and strategies from the pages that follow and success on the NCLEX will become a reality. This approach is innovative, exciting, proven, and extremely user friendly. Use it once; then use it again, and again, and again.

> *Repetition, repetition, repetition* is the key to developing new test-taking behaviors.

ABC: WHAT IT MEANS FOR THE NCLEX

As health care providers we all know what ABC stands for: **A**irway, **B**reathing, and **C**irculation. These are the terms used in cardiopulmonary resuscitation. I propose another meaning for the ABCs that is a key that unlocks many of the secrets of the NCLEX: nurses **A**ssess **B**efore **C**aring and **S**afety. I suggest either manually or visually placing the letters *ABCs* and the corresponding words at the top of every test page or computer screen page before attempting to answer any question. The reason for this is it becomes imperative for the test-taker to think about life-threatening occurrences and/or prioritizing decisions and actions. Once you have visualized or written the ABCs, to the left and to the right envision or write the words "life threatening" and "priority."

The ABCs:

	Airway	**A**	Assess	
Life Threatening	Breathing	**B**	Before	Prioritize
	Circulation	**C**	Caring	
		S	Safety	

Manually write or mentally visualize these terms before reading a question to remind you to choose answers that reflect life-threatening situations and/or priority assessments and interventions.

The item writers for the NCLEX are charged with the responsibility for writing questions that challenge test-takers to prioritize assessments and actions, critically think to problem solve for clients and family members, and demonstrate knowledge of established standards of care. Hence, maintaining a patent **A**irway, fostering adequate **B**reathing movements, and supporting good **C**irculation are the priority interventions for all nurses to keep their clients **S**afe. When any of these priority issues are jeopardized, the client may be placed in a potentially life-threatening situation. To preserve the **S**afety of clients and therefore to meet the standards of care for the profession, a nurse *must* **A**ssess **B**efore **C**aring. In other words, the nurse cannot act or perform *any* intervention before reviewing the situation. This usually ensures the **S**afety of the client. Once a determination is made on the action needed to preserve the physiological safety of the client, then the nurse may intervene.

SUMMARY

As you use this text, keep in mind that the commitment you made to use the techniques you learn and pass the NCLEX on the first try is just pages away. Keep focused, work hard, and be diligent. Now, let's go to work!

The following are testimonials from two of my students who used the 5-Step Approach, skills and strategies, and prepared physically and emotionally for the NCLEX. One is now a registered professional nurse and the second is a new licensed practical nurse.

Student Profile 1

"I was a graduate from nursing school in 1996. I passed the NCLEX-PN on the first try and went to take the NCLEX-RN. On the way to the testing site I experienced an anxiety attack and never tried to go again. In 2005 I met Dr. DiDona through a mutual friend. I worked with Dr. DiDona for 18 months. She taught me to read questions slowly and carefully, to use the 5-Step Approach, 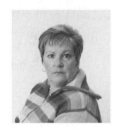 and to use her skills and strategies, including the ABCs of nursing care. I was able to learn how to choose the best answer. I was also able to almost eliminate my anxiety level using the techniques Dr. DiDona taught me. On the day of the test I followed the recommended nutritional suggestions, I did not feel hungry or tired, and I was able to concentrate on my test without experiencing a slump.

"My career goals include one day becoming a nursing instructor or a nurse practitioner. Since I passed my NCLEX-RN examination, I have started

(continues)

(continued)

working as a corrections nurse in a large men's state prison. I am confident in my ability to perform as an RN. If it wasn't for Dr. DiDona building up my confidence using her 5-Step Approach, I might not be where I am today. I know that I will meet my career goals. I encourage all nursing students facing the NCLEX to use this book, learn the techniques, and gain the confidence to be as successful I was!"

Mary Jo Hutchings, RN

Student Profile 2

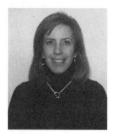

"I met Dr. DiDona through a mutual friend a few years ago. I started private tutoring sessions 1 year later. I worked with Dr. DiDona, learning the 5-Step Approach and using her skills and strategies. I do not think I would have passed the NCLEX without these tools. I have historically always been a poor test taker. Dr. DiDona's skills and strategies and her approach helped me to apply my knowledge. Dr. DiDona always told me to read, read, read! I read everything I could.

"The physiological and psychological preparation Dr. DiDona taught me to follow the day before and the day of the examination was also a tremendous help. I am now working as a licensed practical nurse in a primary care medical office and I am really enjoying my career. I never felt so proud of myself. I have and will continue to recommend Dr. DiDona's 5-Step Approach and her skills and strategies to anyone looking to pass the NCLEX."

Annette DiVenuto-Keefe, LPN

NCLEX-RN TEST PLAN

"The NCLEX-RN Test Plan provides a concise summary of the content and scope of the licensing examination. It serves as a guide for examination development as well as candidate preparation" (National Council of State Boards of Nursing [NCSBN], 2007, p. 1). Understanding the NCLEX-RN test plan is an important part of preparing to test. The test plan demonstrates the structure and framework involved in creating every question. The test plan also provides a universal configuration in the cataloging of acceptable nursing assessments, interventions, and competencies while referencing clients and families in a wide variety of health care settings. The parts of the test plan are divided into two major categories, and although intertwined in the formation of the test plan, each is discussed in the next sections separately from one other. The first category is Client Needs and the second category is Integrated Processes.

Client Needs

There are four main Client Needs categories, two of which are further subdivided. As observed over the years and confirmed by past testers, I present the four categories in order of importance as follows:

- Physiological Integrity
    - Basic Care and Comfort
    - Pharmacological and Parenteral Therapies
    - Reduction of Risk Potential
    - Physiological Adaptation
- Psychosocial Integrity
- Safe and Effective Care Environment
    - Management of Care
    - Safety and Infection Control
- Health Promotion and Maintenance

Integrated Processes

There are four processes identified by the NCSBN that are an integral part of the NCLEX-RN test plan and are interwoven into the Client Needs categories and subcategories throughout the NCLEX-RN examination structure. In 2007 the NCSBN defined these processes as follows:

- *Nursing Process:* A scientific problem-solving approach to client care that includes assessment, analysis, planning, implementation, and evaluation.
- *Caring:* Interaction of the nurse and client in an atmosphere of mutual respect and trust. In this collaborative environment the nurse provides encouragement, hope, support, and compassion to help achieve desired outcomes.
- *Communication and Documentation:* Verbal and nonverbal interactions between the nurse and client, the client's significant others, and the other members of the health care team. Events and activities associated with client care are validated in written and/or electronic records that reflect standards of practice and accountability in the provision of care.
- *Teaching/Learning:* Facilitation of the acquisition of knowledge, skills, and attitudes promoting a change in behavior (NCSBN, 2007, p. 3).

Overview of Content

The Client Needs categories and subcategories cover the life span of clients and family members and are further defined on the following page. The content relative to each category is presented in an abbreviated design.

Physiological Integrity: Protection and Safety

■ *Basic Care and Comfort:* Palliative Care, Personal Hygiene, Elimination, Mobility, Comfort Measures, Rest, Nutrition, Hydration

■ *Pharmacological and Parenteral Therapies:* Adverse Reactions, Blood Administration, Calculation of Dosage and Intravenous Fluids, Actions and Outcomes, Pain Management

■ *Reduction of Risk Potential:* Diagnostic Testing, Treatments and Procedures, Body System/Health Alterations, Vital Signs

■ *Physiological Adaptation:* Fluids and Electrolytes, Emergency Events, Responses to Therapies, Illness Management, Infectious Diseases

Psychosocial Integrity: Mental Well-Being

■ Religious and Spiritual Needs, Alterations in Sensory and Perceptual Needs, Coping With Stress, Cultural Differences/Preferences, Grief and Loss, Mental Health Issues, Dealing With a Crisis, Negative Behavioral Attributes, Significant Others/Support Systems Changes, Therapeutic Communication

Safe and Effective Care Environment: Enhancement and Protection

■ *Management of Care:* Management and Practice, Patient Rights, Confidentiality, Collaboration, Consultation and Resource Allocation, Informed Consent, Legal Issues, Education and Supervision of Staff, Advocacy

■ *Safety and Infection Control:* Asepsis and Sterility Maintenance, Incident Reporting, Fall and Injury Prevention, Proper Handling and Disposal of Hazardous Material, Disaster Planning, Safe Use of Equipment/Restraints

Health Promotion and Maintenance: Detection and Development

■ Screening Programs, Risk Reduction, Self-Care, Physical Assessment, Principles of Growth and Development, Health and Wellness, Prevention of Illness, Immunizations, Aging, Human Sexuality

NCLEX-PN TEST PLAN

"The entry-level practical/vocational nurse demonstrates the essential competencies needed to care for clients with commonly occurring health problems that have predictable outcomes" (NCSBN, 2005, p. 2). The importance of understanding the NCLEX-PN test plan cannot be understated. The test reflects skills and knowledge that are considered vital for the practical/vocational nurse to possess. The NCLEX-PN test plan serves as a "how to" manual for the construction of questions for item writers and as a blueprint for schools of nursing to develop curriculum for candidate preparation. The parts of the NCLEX-PN test plan are also divided into two major categories and are discussed separately in the next sections. It is important to remember that these categories interconnect in the formation of the examination questions. The first category is Client Needs, and the second category is Integrated Processes.

Client Needs

There are four main Client Needs categories. Two of these categories are further subdivided. These areas were selected to be representative of the scope of practice for the practical/vocational nurse. Over the years of teaching students to prepare for the NCLEX-PN, it has come to my attention that there is a priority in the ranking of the Client Needs as follows:

- Physiological Integrity
  - Basic Care and Comfort
  - Pharmacological Therapies
  - Reduction of Risk Potential
  - Physiological Adaptation
- Psychosocial Integrity
- Safe and Effective Care Environment
  - Coordinated Care
  - Safety and Infection Control
- Health Promotion and Maintenance

Integrated Processes

There are four processes identified by the NCSBN that are considered essential components of the NCLEX-PN test plan and are interlaced into the Client Needs categories and subcategories. In 2005 the NCSBN defined these processes as follows:

- *Clinical Problem-Solving Process (Nursing Process):* A scientific approach to client care that includes data collection, planning, implementation, and evaluation.

- *Caring:* Interaction of the practical/vocational nurse and clients, families, and significant others in an atmosphere of mutual respect and trust. In this collaborative environment the practical/vocational nurse provides support and compassion to help achieve desired therapeutic outcomes.

- *Communication and Documentation:* Verbal and nonverbal interactions between the practical/vocational nurse and clients, families, significant others, and members of the health care team. Events and activities associated with client care are validated in written and/or electronic records that reflect standards of practice and accountability in the provision of care.

- *Teaching and Learning:* Facilitation of the acquisition of knowledge, skills, and attitudes to assist in promoting positive changes in behavior (NCSBN, 2005, p. 3).

Overview of Content

The Client Needs categories and subcategories are presented here in an abbreviated format. The content, defined on the following page, covers the life span of clients and family members. The list presented is not inclusive but rather a sampling of the major components of the test plan.

Physiological Integrity: Health and Well-Being

- *Basic Care and Comfort:* Nutrition, Hydration, Hygiene, Mobility, Rest and Sleep
- *Pharmacological Therapies:* Side Effects, Agents and Actions, Adverse Reactions, Predictable Outcomes
- *Reduction of Risk Potential:* Vital Signs, Testing, Treatments and Procedures
- *Physiological Adaptation:* Pathophysiology, Emergencies, Therapies and Responses

Psychosocial Integrity: Mental Well-Being

- Crisis Intervention, Stress Management, Therapeutic Communication, Grief and Loss, Coping Strategies, Abuse, Spiritual Issues, Suicide and Violence Safety Measures, Support Systems, Management of Behaviors

Safe and Effective Care Environment: Enhancement and Protection

- *Coordinated Care:* Advocacy, Informed Consent, Ethical Issues, Legal Issues, Confidentiality, Rights and Responsibilities
- *Safety and Infection Control:* Restraints/Safety Devices, Incident Reporting, Appropriate Use of Equipment, Accident and Injury Prevention, Asepsis and Sterility Topics

Health Promotion and Maintenance: Development and Prevention

- Normal Aging, Immunizations, Screening Programs, Lifestyle Issues and Self-Care, Prevention of Disease, Family Planning

It is important to remember that knowing the NCLEX test plan, and understanding the role it plays in guiding item writers, will assist the test-taker in eliminating distracters and home in on the right answer. Study the test plan, become familiar with the components, and recognize that this knowledge is an essential part of your overall transformation to becoming a successful test-taker.

REFERENCES

National Council of State Boards of Nursing. (2005). *NCLEX-PN test plan.* Retrieved January 11, 2008, from https://www.ncsbn.org/PN_test_plan_05_Web.pdf

National Council of State Boards of Nursing. (2007). *NCLEX-RN test plan.* Retrieved January 11, 2008, from https://www.ncsbn.org/RN_Test_Plan_2007_Web.pdf

As discussed in Chapter 1, test-taking skills and strategies are extremely important tools that can aid the test-taker in uncovering the correct answer to a question. This chapter discusses specific skills and strategies, presents the types of questions that lend themselves to applying these tools, and includes sample questions for the reader to practice applying his or her newly acquired test-taking skills and strategies.

SKILLS AND STRATEGIES

I have studied the skills and strategies to be discussed in this chapter for over 17 years. Applying the principles behind these tools has, over time, proven to be 90% to 95% effective for test-takers. As there is rarely an "always," there is constantly room for exceptions in testing situations. But if these tools are learned and applied, the test-taker should have a better than average chance of choosing the correct answer. Your accuracy for guessing the answer to a question will increase from 50% to 60% up to 90% to 95%!

Example Questions and Rationales

Each skill and strategy presented here will be applicable 90% to 95% of the time. Nothing is ever 100% for sure. If learned and practiced with intent and dedication, NCLEX success will be knocking at your door.

> The skills and strategies will help the test-taker find the right answer 90% to 95% of the time.

In this section, a skill or strategy is presented and then an example question, answer, and rationale follow.

STRATEGY

Never choose an answer that contains the following words: *always, never, all,* and *only*. These words do not allow for the possibility of an exception, and therefore the answers that contain these words can be automatically eliminated.

EXAMPLE QUESTION:

Elderly clients who experience depression present with needs different from younger adults in that in the elderly

1. Symptoms of other illnesses may mask sadness.
2. Cognitive impairment is never present.
3. Psychosomatic symptoms always take over.
4. All traditional antidepressant medications are useless methods of treatment.

Answer: 1

Rationale: Answers 2, 3, and 4 contain the words *never*, *always*, and *all*, and do not allow for any exceptions.

STRATEGY

Never choose an answer that describes the nurse's actions as "vigorous." Nurses seldom perform interventions vigorously. Discard answers using this word.

EXAMPLE QUESTION:

The nurse is caring for a client with second- and third-degree burns. Hydrotherapy is ordered daily. The nurse knows that the purpose of hydrotherapy includes all the following *except*

1. Gentle debridement of dead tissue.
2. Stimulation of circulation.
3. Vigorous massaging of nonburned areas.
4. Increase in the rate of healing.

Answer: 3

Rationale: Vigorous actions are not part of the nurse's interventions.

STRATEGY

Do not pass the buck. Professional registered nurses (RNs) seldom pass a nursing problem off to the doctor. An RN always attempts to critically think and problem solve. This is especially true in areas that address questions from clients regarding care or procedures. Look for the answers that use the nurse's aptitude to assess and deduce. The same holds true for the practical/vocational nurse (LPN). He or she should always try to problem solve within the scope of LPN practice before calling on the charge nurse for assistance.

EXAMPLE QUESTION:

A 30-year-old female client diagnosed with invasive breast cancer must start chemotherapy. She tells the nurse she is worried about the side effects of the treatments. The nurse's best response would be which if the following?

1. "I will have your doctor discuss the side effects with you."
2. "I will have a representative from the American Cancer Association come to see you soon."
3. "What is it about the side effects that worry you?"
4. "Would you like to speak to your oncologist before starting the treatments?"

Answer: 3

Rationale: The nurse takes responsibility for answering the client's concerns as an initial intervention.

STRATEGY

Hand washing is an important action for all nurses in all situations. Item writers for the NCLEX typically agree with this belief and usually manage to put a few questions about hand washing into the NCLEX test bank. Unless *glaringly* wrong, choose the answer that directs the nurse to wash his or her hands.

EXAMPLE QUESTION:

Nurses know that the best way of preventing the spread of disease is to

1. Properly dispose of used tissues.
2. Discard used syringes in appropriate containers.
3. Change soiled linens daily for clients with draining wounds.
4. Wash hands frequently and consistently.

Answer: 4

Rationale: Hand washing is the best way of preventing the spread of microorganisms and should always be considered the priority action.

> **STRATEGY**
>
> **When considering questions that deal with nurses communicating with clients, the item writers typically look for the test-taker to choose the answer that demonstrates the nurse *empathizing* with the client. Hence, steer clear of answers that contain the following words or that imply the following meanings: judge(s), confront(s), argue(s), challenge(s), insist(s), and question(s). Also, never choose an answer that contains punitive language on the nurse's part, such as the phrase "or else."**

EXAMPLE QUESTION:

A family member is arguing with the nurse over the client's diet order. The family member wants to bring in food not included in the client's diet. The nurse knows that proper nutrition is necessary for healing and for the general well-being of the client. What should be the nurse's priority action?

1. Ask the family member why he wants to hurt the client's chances of healing.
2. Confront the family member on his knowledge of the food pyramid.

3. Report the family member's ridiculous request to the doctor as soon as possible.
4. Discuss with the family member the foods allowed on the diet and ways to incorporate some favorite items.

Answer: 4

Rationale: Answers 1, 2, and 3 do not foster communication or trust and may make the family member and client feel uncomfortable.

STRATEGY

Frequently, answers contain multiple parts. It is important to remember that *all* components of an answer must be correct. There is no such answer that is partially right. It is *entirely correct or it is not the answer*.

EXAMPLE QUESTION:

A nurse is preparing to administer a soap-water enema to the client. Which nursing intervention is correct for the nurse to perform?

1. Put on sterile gloves and turn the client to the left Sims' position.
2. Check the temperature of the water solution to ensure it is between 90°F and 95°F and hang the container 18 inches above the client's rectum.
3. Lubricate the end of the tubing and insert it at least 8 inches.
4. Administer the fluid slowly and stop the flow of solution if the client complains of cramps.

Answer: 4

Rationale: Gloves do not need to be sterile. The water temperature should be between 100°F and 105°F. The tube should only be inserted 4 inches. Answer 4 has all correct parts.

STRATEGY Questions often refer to the health and well-being of clients. For these questions, look for answers that teach or encourage the client to *avoid using alcohol, caffeine, and tobacco.* Nurses seldom encourage clients to limit usage of these products.

EXAMPLE QUESTION:

A 35-week pregnant primigravida comes to the clinic for her routine check-up. She tells the nurse that she is going to a New Year's Eve party at a neighbor's home the next day. She also states that this annual gala has a reputation of being loud and smoky, and food and alcohol are plentiful. What health teaching regarding the well-being of the fetus is *best* for the nurse to offer?

1. "You should avoid drinking any alcohol and breathing in any smoke."
2. "You should limit your alcohol consumption to a champagne toast at midnight."
3. "Second-hand smoke will not hurt you or the baby."
4. "Having wine with dinner should satisfy your need to drink."

Answer: 1

Rationale: There is no alcohol or nicotine consumption recommended during pregnancy. Nurses do not suggest limiting exposure to or ingestion of teratogens. There is evidence in the literature that second-hand smoke does cause harm.

STRATEGY There are usually questions on the nutritional value of foods on the NCLEX-RN and -PN. When you come across a question that is about the *nutritional value* of food, always choose the answer that contains *chicken.* It is high in protein for healing, and it is low in fat for health. This makes it a prime choice for a healthy food.

EXAMPLE QUESTION:

An obese client with poor peripheral circulation is suffering from a lower leg ulcer. Which of the following food choices is best to promote wound healing and support weight loss?

1. BLT sandwich on whole-wheat toast, low-fat mayo, fruit-flavored sherbet, and decaf coffee.
2. Cheeseburger, French fries, fruit ice, and a diet soda.
3. Grilled chicken on a half-roll, carrot salad, and skim milk.
4. Scrambled eggs, lean bacon, buttered muffin, and tea.

Answer: 3

Rationale: Answers 1 and 4 have bacon, a fatty source of protein. Answer 2 is also high in fats. Chicken is lean and a good source of protein. The caloric content of answer #3 is also the lowest.

STRATEGY

When a client communicates with the nurse, the nurse is duty bound to foster that communication. When you answer questions about client–nurse communications, always choose the answer that *encourages, allows, and promotes verbalization* on the client's part. Also, select answers that show the nurse using open-ended questions. Never choose the answer that requires a "yes" or "no" reply from the client. Look for answers that have the nurse using phrases such as "Tell me more" and "Let's discuss/talk about. . . ." The answer that has the client giving information is usually right.

EXAMPLE QUESTION:

The parents of a 4-year-old child recently diagnosed with a chronic illness are discussing the changes they have made in the home to properly care for their child. The mother states that they have moved the child's bed into their room, have fired their baby-sitter because they will not need to go out any longer, and have taken their child's name off the list for Little League baseball for the spring. Which statement by the nurse fosters therapeutic communication with these parents?

1. "Was your babysitter incompetent?"
2. "Do you feel more comfortable with your child sleeping in your room?"
3. "Baseball is considered a very dangerous sport."
4. "Tell me more about the changes you have made."

Answer: 4

Rationale: Answers 1, 2, and 3 do not invite any discussion with the parents. Answer 4 encourages the parents to continue giving information.

STRATEGY

When reading answers to questions that discuss the client directly, look for the answer that *personalizes or individualizes the information*. Avoid answers that generalize or globalize the situation. Assessments and cares should be *customized* to the client and not to the general population.

EXAMPLE QUESTION:

A client suffering from moderate anxiety is pacing the hall and mumbling. As the nurse approaches the client he states, "I am at the end of my rope. I don't think I can take any more bad news." Which of the following statements made by the nurse is best *initially*?

1. "Most clients like you benefit from lying down."
2. "Come with me to a private area where we can talk without interruption."
3. "Doctors usually recommend relaxation exercises for client's who are as upset as you are."
4. "An antianxiety pill works best for situations like this."

Answer: 2

Rationale: Answers 1, 3, and 4 do not address the client as an individual but generalizes the client's symptoms. Answer 2 personalizes the nurse's actions to the client.

STRATEGY

Every so often you find questions that seem easy or obvious. These questions may make you doubt your understanding of the question. I call these questions "ah-ha" moments. When you are deep into the test and concentrating with all your ability and one of these questions presents, you may suddenly find your concentration broken. This "ah-ha" moment is a gift, and I strongly urge you to take advantage of it. Sit up, stretch, take a few deep breaths, and go back to work. These opportunities are refreshing and rejuvenating and can clear away any mental cobwebs that may have formed during the testing time, so use them wisely.

EXAMPLE QUESTION:

A postoperative client is complaining of incisional pain. The physician has ordered morphine SQ. Before administering this medication, the nurse should complete which priority assessment?

1. Blood pressure.
2. Apical heart rate.
3. Respiratory rate.
4. Temperature.

Answer: 3 (ah-ha!)

Rationale: Remembering Airway, Breathing, and Circulation will certainly guide your choice here. Enjoy the moment and refresh yourself. Take a deep breath and stretch!

> Take advantage of "ah-ha" moments and refresh yourself.

STRATEGY

Avoid answers that question a client about his or her feelings, negate one's feelings, or tell the client how to feel. Feelings are personal and should be respected.

EXAMPLE QUESTION:

A woman, whose mother suffered a cerebral vascular accident and has right-sided paralysis and aphasia, is upset and tells the nurse she knows her mother will never be the same. She also tells the nurse she feels responsible for her mother's condition because she did not force her aging mother to come live with her. Which of the following responses by the nurse would be *best*?

1. "Tell me more about what you are feeling."
2. "Your mother will be fine. Don't worry so much."
3. "You could not have prevented the stroke."
4. "You are not responsible for your aging mother."

Answer: 1

Rationale: Answers 2, 3, and 4 tell the woman that her feelings are wrong or do not matter. Answer 1 demonstrates interest and caring on the part of the nurse, and shows respect for how the daughter is feeling.

STRATEGY

When answers seem similar to each other and you consider them to be correct answers, choose the one option that gives the most information. Very often in situations like this, at least two answers contain identical data but one contains some extra data. Select the answer that gives the most details. In other words, choose the answer that is the *most comprehensive, all-inclusive, or detailed*.

EXAMPLE QUESTION:

A nurse is helping an elderly client to ambulate in the hallway for the first time. The client has brought her walker from home. To ensure proper use of the walker and the safety of the client, the nurse should

1. Walk closely behind the client.
2. Walk in front of the client, helping to move the walker.
3. Walk to the side of the client.
4. Walk close behind and to the side of the client.

Answer: 4

Rationale: Although answers 1 and 3 could be considered correct, answer 4 is more inclusive. Therefore 4 is the better answer.

STRATEGY

Avoid answers that portray the nurse as someone who is giving excuses for events out of his or her realm of responsibility. Some examples include the nurse accepting accountability for bad-tasting or inappropriate foods, inadequate supportive care, and uncomfortable linen. Look for the answer that has the nurse referring the client to the appropriate resource or has the nurse contacting the appropriate person(s) directly to address the problem.

EXAMPLE QUESTION:

A client calls the nurse into his room and bitterly complains about certain aspects of his care and his hospital stay. Which response by the nurse would be appropriate in addressing the client's concerns?

1. "I agree. The food here is not very good since the new chef arrived."
2. "The laundry room needs to use fabric softeners to make the sheets softer."
3. "I will have the housekeeping manager come to speak to you about your dirty bathroom."
4. "I'm sorry the therapist was rude to you. Their client load is very big."

Answer: 3

Rationale: Answers 1, 2, and 4 show the nurse taking on the responsibility or making excuses when other departments fall short of expectations. Answer 3 refers the correct personnel directly to the client to discuss the issues.

When a question is describing the signs and symptoms a client is exhibiting, routinely the *first* symptom mentioned in the question is considered to be the priority. There is often intent or purpose in the order in which things are listed. The answer chosen should address that first symptom.

EXAMPLE QUESTION:

A 54-year-old man comes to the emergency room complaining of severe crushing chest pain after playing a round of golf. His vital signs are pulse 104, respirations 26, and blood pressure 160/100. The physician orders morphine sulfate 10 mg SQ stat, cardiac monitoring, oxygen 2 L via nasal cannula, electrocardiogram, cardiac enzymes, and an IV 5% dextrose and normal saline at a KVO rate. What is the nurse's priority intervention?

1. Administer the morphine.
2. Administer the oxygen.
3. Connect the cardiac monitor.
4. Draw the blood for cardiac enzymes.

Answer: 1

Rationale: Although all the doctor's orders are important, the nurse must address the severe crushing chest pain. Pain may be a factor in keeping the client's vital signs elevated. Pain is also the first symptom referenced in the question.

> The first symptom referenced in a question is usually the priority and should be addressed initially.

STRATEGY

More often than not, remembering Airway, Breathing, and Circulation will guide you to the correct answer. In addition to the ABCs being a viable solution to a question, it has also been noted that frequently when *infection* is offered as an option, it is the correct answer (approximately 75% of the time). The seriousness of the infection should also be considered by the test-taker.

EXAMPLE QUESTION:

A toddler has been diagnosed with acute nephrotic syndrome. The nurse is teaching the mother about important changes and signs and symptoms to report to the physician. Which of the following is most important to report to the physician?

1. Sneezing and discolored nasal discharge.
2. Fatigue and irritability.
3. Poor appetite and increased thirst.
4. Swelling of the face and hands.

Answer: 1

Rationale: Answer 1 suggests the possibility of an infection. Answers 2, 3, and 4 are important but expected symptoms for the child with nephritic syndrome. Therefore, they should not be considered as priorities.

STRATEGY

As a nurse comes upon a situation, his or her first assessments or interventions should be directed toward the client. The client is typically the priority, followed by family members, equipment, and then the environment.

EXAMPLE QUESTION:

A nurse is making morning rounds and finds a client who is 4 days post-op sitting in a chair and visiting with his wife. The client states he is hungry and wants to brush his teeth. His wife tells you she needs to meet with the social worker to make arrangements to take her husband home tomorrow. The client's dinner tray from last night is sitting on an empty chair and his incentive spirometer is out of his reach on the window ledge. What would be the nurse's priority intervention?

1. Offer the client his incentive spirometer to use.
2. Call the social worker to come and meet with the wife.
3. Remove the old dinner tray from the room.
4. Allow the client to brush his teeth and order a breakfast tray.

Answer: 4

Rationale: Answer 4 addresses the physiological needs the client has requested be met. The social worker can then be contacted for the wife and the room organized. A client 4 days post-op and ambulating does not require an incentive spirometer.

STRATEGY

Try to stay away from the urge to say to yourself "What if . . ." or "Suppose. . . ." Reading into questions is never a good idea and often leads to the wrong answer. The questions have all the information you need to know. There are no "trick" questions. The item writers cannot give you less information than you need to answer the question, but they can give you more. Learning to sift through the unimportant information takes practice.

EXAMPLE QUESTION:

A client diagnosed with diabetes mellitus is admitted to your unit. The client has been taking insulin for 3 years and is considered controlled with a normal A1C level. The client has a cellulitis of the left great toe from cutting his own toenails. It is draining clear fluid from a small opening near the nail bed. His temperature is 101.2°F, pulse 98, respirations 24, and blood pressure 130/82. His fingerstick glucose is 112, and his white blood cell count is elevated. When caring for this client, the nurse should remember that

1. Clients with normal A1C levels are at greater risk for developing episodes of hypoglycemia.
2. Diabetics with elevated white blood cell counts always have blood cultures drawn immediately.
3. It is important to practice universal precautions when caring for this client.
4. It is vital that this client's fingerstick glucose levels be monitored every 3 hours.

Answer: 3

Rationale: This question simply wanted the test-taker to apply safe standards of care. That is, all clients are to be treated with universal precautions. Answers 1, 2, and 4 are not true.

STRATEGY

Some questions ask for what I call "negative" responses. These questions use phrases such as "The nurse would *not* do . . ."; "The nurse would *not* assess . . ."; ". . . *all but which* . . ."; "The nurse/client would/should *avoid* . . ."; and "The nurse/client is *least likely*. . . ." The test-taker must be alert to these words and phrases and remember to read the question carefully to completely understand what is being asked.

EXAMPLE QUESTION:

A new mother is breastfeeding her infant and asks about her dietary needs. You know she has many food allergies and sensitivities. The nurse tells the mother to avoid all of the following foods *except*

1. Peanuts.
2. Shellfish.
3. Beef.
4. Eggs.

Answer: 3

Rationale: Answers 1, 2, and 4 are known to cause allergic reactions. Beef has the least chance of causing an allergic response. (See Chapter 4.)

STRATEGY

Unless contraindicated by the surgical procedure itself, select the answer that offers the position of choice for postoperative clients as *low Fowler's*. This position facilitates lung expansion and decreases pressure on the vena cava.

EXAMPLE QUESTION:

A client returns from the post–anesthesia care unit after a cholecystectomy. The recovery room nurse reports that the vital signs are stable and the dressing is clean and dry. The client has not voided. After placing the client in bed, the nurse adjusts the height of the head of the bed to

1. High Fowler's to facilitate rest.
2. Low Fowler's to decrease pressure on the vena cava.
3. Left lateral to decrease pressure on the incision.
4. Reverse Trendelenburg to decrease intracranial pressure.

Answer: 2

Rationale: Unless the client has had back surgery or spinal anesthesia, low Fowler's up to semi-Fowler's is desirable. Remember, post-op clients need to cough and deep breathe and frequently suffer from nausea. This position not only allows complete expansion of the lungs, it is safest to avoid aspiration of vomitus.

STRATEGY

When referring to medical diagnoses that are *progressive in nature* and asking about *early* signs and symptoms of the disease progression, choose "fatigue" as the answer. Fatigue is often the earliest sign that illness is threatening or has begun.

EXAMPLE QUESTION:

A client newly diagnosed with rheumatoid arthritis tells the nurse she came to the clinic initially because she observed which of the following *early* sign of the disease?

1. Fatigue.
2. Pain in her feet.
3. Swelling of her joints.
4. Morning stiffness.

Answer: 1

Rationale: Fatigue is often the earliest sign of disease onset. Physiological changes happen over time and therefore occur later.

Conversely, when referring to medical diagnoses that are *progressive in nature* and asking about *late* signs and symptoms of the disease progression, choose the answer that reflects *advanced physiological changes and/or deformities*. These changes typically occur over a period of time and are therefore not seen until the disease is advanced.

EXAMPLE QUESTION:

A client comes to the clinic for a routine evaluation. She was diagnosed with rheumatoid arthritis 2 years ago. She is complaining of increasing pain and stiffness in her hands, especially in the morning. Upon physical examination the nurse would expect to see which of the following?

1. Thinning of the fingers.
2. Deformities of the knuckles.
3. Increased range of motion in the thumbs.
4. Lack of blanching in the nail beds.

Answer: 2

Rationale: Answers 1, 3, and 4 are not physiological changes associated with rheumatoid arthritis. Joint deformities are a late sign of the disease progression.

STRATEGY

As stated previously, nurses Assess Before Caring. Hence, when faced with questions that ask the test-taker to determine what the nurse does initially, always remember to choose the answer that *assesses what the client knows and assesses the situation*.

EXAMPLE QUESTION:

The physician has prescribed nitroglycerin tablets sublingually to a client newly diagnosed with angina pectoris. The client asks the nurse how long he has to take the medication before his condition is cured. The nurse should first

1. Ask the client what he knows about his diagnosis.
2. Make sure the client knows how to correctly take his medication.
3. Provide the client with written information about angina pectoris.
4. Reassure the client that his condition will improve with medication compliance.

Answer: 1

Rationale: The nurse assesses first and foremost. Understanding what the client knows about the diagnosis is the priority for meeting his needs. Answers 2 and 3 ignore the client's concerns, and answer 4 is incorrect.

STRATEGY | **Never select an answer where the nurse gives his or her opinion. Nurses provide information that allows clients to make informed decisions, but nurses by no means offer advice.**

EXAMPLE QUESTION:

A newly delivered mother of three tells the nurse she does not want any more children and asks what method of birth control the nurse would recommend. The nurse would correctly respond by saying which of the following?

1. "I prefer to take birth control pills. I think they are the most reliable."
2. "Your doctor usually recommends using a diaphragm and spermicidal cream."
3. "Having your doctor place an intrauterine device into your uterus will eliminate your worry regarding pregnancy."
4. "You are concerned about getting pregnant again."

Answer: 4

Rationale: Answers 1, 2, and 3 do not provide the client with any knowledge about available birth control methods and demonstrate the nurse giving advice. Answer 4 encourages the client to talk and can lead to an assessment of her knowledge of birth control methods.

STRATEGY

To answer questions that ask for information regarding client care after leaving the hospital, always choose the answer that includes rehabilitation planning and/or discharge planning. And remember, rehabilitation and discharge planning always *begin on the day of admission*.

EXAMPLE QUESTION:

A 78-year-old man is admitted to the intensive care unit after a cerebral vascular accident. He has left-sided weakness, an unstable blood pressure, and a low-grade fever. His elderly wife tells the nurse she is worried and confused as to the treatment protocol for her husband. The correct response by the nurse is which of the following?

1. "We have begun plans to discharge your husband to a rehabilitation facility as soon as he is stable."
2. "Your husband is too critical to consider what tomorrow will bring. Let's just concentrate on today."
3. "Don't worry. Most clients like your husband have no residual effects after a few days of rest."
4. "You will have to speak to the doctor for that information."

Answer: 1

Rationale: Answers 2, 3, and 4 are unrealistic or untrue. Answer 1 directly addresses the wife's concern and demonstrates that discharge and rehabilitation planning begin on admission.

STRATEGY

Avoid selecting answers that use the words *complete, total,* and *exclusively*. These answers do not allow for the possibility of an exception.

EXAMPLE QUESTION:

The nurse is teaching a client newly diagnosed with diabetes mellitus how to administer his insulin and to eat a healthy and balanced diet. The client tells the nurse that he has a brother who also has diabetes and who has taught him what foods he can and cannot eat. Which statement made by the client indicates to the nurse the need for *further* teaching?

1. "My brother knows to rotate his injection sites every day."
2. "I know I must follow a diet that completely eliminates bread and pasta."
3. "It is important that I do not shake the insulin vial but just roll it in my hand."
4. "Graham crackers are a good bedtime snack for me to have."

Answer: 2

Rationale: Answers 1, 3, and 4 are all positive and true statements, and demonstrate learning has taken place. Answer 2 is untrue and contains the word *completely*. Did you use numbering or 1 B and 3 Gs? (See Chapter 4.)

STRATEGY

Avoid choosing answers that include the phrases "large meals" and "mega-doses of vitamins or medications." It is seldom recommended that clients ingest large or significant quantities of food or drugs.

EXAMPLE QUESTION:

A client with gastroesophageal reflux disease complains to the nurse that he suffers with severe pyrexia every night. The nurse assesses the client's bedtime habits and discovers the following contributing factor:

1. The client sleeps with the head of his bed slightly elevated.
2. The client takes his prescribed medication every night as directed by the physician.
3. The client sleeps in the left lateral position as much as possible.
4. The client works late hours and usually has a large dinner before going to bed.

Answer: 4

Rationale: Eating a large meal before retiring for the night is not recommended. If the client must eat before bedtime, a small light dinner is best. Answers 1, 2, and 3 are positive actions to prevent episodes of gastroesophageal reflux disease.

STRATEGY **"Quackery" is a term that has appeared in review questions in the recent past. Do not select answers that include this term because it is misleading and insulting to the beliefs of the client and family.**

EXAMPLE QUESTION:

A client shows the nurse her copper bracelet and explains that it helps her to feel better. The nurse would correctly respond with all the following comments *except*

1. "I am glad you feel better wearing your bracelet."
2. "Tell me more about how you are feeling."

3. "Believing objects have powers to make you feel better is quackery. Let me explain how your medicine helps you to feel better."

4. "Do you wear the bracelet all the time or just when you have pain?"

Answer: 3

Rationale: The nurse demonstrates knowledge that the bracelet is harmless for the client in answers 1, 2, and 4. Answer 3 is insulting and judgmental.

When questions describe multiple problems for the client, the signs and symptoms that are stated as "new onset" should be treated as the priority assessment for the nurse. Hence, choose the answer that addresses these dilemmas.

EXAMPLE QUESTION:

A client with a history of myocardial infarction comes to the emergency department complaining of bilateral calf pain. He states that it began 2 weeks ago when he began a more advanced stretching and exercise regimen. The client also states that he has been experiencing a new onset of indigestion for the past 24 hours. The nurse's priority assessment should include which of the following?

1. Further questioning the client regarding his complaint of indigestion.
2. Getting an electrocardiogram stat.
3. Applying a warm moist wrap to the client's lower legs.
4. Requesting the lab to draw cardiac enzymes and thrombin level.

Answer: 1

Rationale: Answer 1 is an assessment of the new onset complaint. Answers 2, 3, and 4 are interventions that address issues that are important but are not new and are nonacute.

STRATEGY

Answers that include an instruction to have the client "avoid direct sunlight" are typically the correct answer. This is due to reactions clients have to certain medications when exposed to direct sunlight and to the general belief that direct sunlight can cause harmful skin irritations.

EXAMPLE QUESTION:

The nurse is teaching a client being treated after breast cancer about taking the drug tamoxifen. Which comment by the client indicates teaching has been effective?

1. "I will only be on this medication for 6 months."
2. "As long as I take my medication daily I do not have to see my oncologist."
3. "I am going to the beach for a few days and will take my beach umbrella to sit under every day."
4. "I do not need any blood work as long as I am on the medication."

Answer: 3

Rationale: Tamoxifen is taken for 5 years. Regular visits to the oncologist and screening of client's blood work are necessary. Sun bathing is discouraged due to photophobia. Did you use Bs and Gs? Also, step 4 would apply as answer #3 is the longest or step 5 would work (see Chapter 4).

STRATEGY

In the *absence* of physiological problems and complaints in the question, stress is a better than average choice as a cause of a client's troubles.

EXAMPLE QUESTION:

At 1 a.m. a client is found pacing the hallway of an acute care setting. When approached by the night nurse he states that he "feels fine physically." The nurse assesses the client and finds his vital signs within the normal range. When asked about his inability to sleep, which answer, if given by the client, is the best indication of why the client is awake?

1. "My wife has done a great job handling the house and kids while I have been here."
2. "My boss called today and told me he was going to replace me at work but that it would probably only be a temporary change."
3. "My doctor said that my blood work results were better than they have been in years."
4. "My oldest son was accepted into college and received a sports scholarship."

Answer: 2

Rationale: Answers 1, 3, and 4 are positive stresses. Answer 2 is worrisome for a man to feel his means of supporting his family is at risk.

STRATEGY

When physical needs for clients are discussed in the question, always choose the answer that focuses directly on these physical requirements.

EXAMPLE QUESTION:

A client is admitted to the step-down unit after a motor vehicle accident. He is complaining of generalized pain from injuries suffered when his car was struck. The physician has ordered Demerol for pain, admission blood work, an electrocardiogram, regular diet, out of bed with assistance, and physical therapy consult. Which action by the nurse should be the priority?

1. Request the electrocardiogram be done stat.
2. Call the lab to come and draw blood.
3. Send a request form to physical therapy.
4. Medicate the client for pain.

Answer: 4

Rationale: Although all orders by the physician must be completed, the client has only one complaint. That is, pain, and therefore administration of Demerol is the priority.

STRATEGY

Pay close attention to questions that discuss time frames for clients to take medication at home. Clients should be instructed to take medication on time but also on a schedule that is convenient.

EXAMPLE QUESTION:

A cardiac client is being discharged home with multiple prescriptions for medication. The nurse is completing discharge teaching, which includes instructions on taking the medications at appropriate times when at home. Which comment by the nurse is **best**?

1. "I understand you do not think taking your medications at the same time as you have in the hospital is convenient, but you cannot change the schedule we have for you."
2. "Let's work out a time schedule that is convenient for you on a daily basis."
3. "You will have to get your doctors approval to change the times of your medications."
4. "It doesn't really matter what time you take your medications as long as you don't skip any doses."

Answer: 2

Rationale: Client compliance with medication is the priority. The nurse should assist the client in taking his medication on time and on a schedule that meets his needs. Answers 1 and 3 are argumentative. Answer 4 is not true.

STRATEGY **When the question refers to future events, is it usually safe to choose the answer that reflects Psychosocial Integrity, because the client is probably worried about the outcome of that event.**

EXAMPLE QUESTION:

A client with benign prostatic hypertrophy is admitted for surgery. The nurse is completing the admission assessment form when the client states, "I don't know what I will do if they find I have cancer." The nurse's best interpretation of this statement is which of the following?

1. The client is experiencing scrotal pain he cannot explain.
2. The client wants to be alone in a private room.
3. The client is fearful of being incapacitated by or dying from cancer.
4. The client is worried about being out of work for a week or so.

Answer: 3

Rationale: Fear of the unknown is a powerful emotion. The client is worried that the doctors may find something wrong with him that will greatly impact his life. There is no indication he is experiencing pain or wants a private room. The client does not mention work.

STRATEGY **When deciding what should be the nurse's priority action or nursing intervention, first eliminate the actions that are appropriate for a nursing assistant or unlicensed assistive personnel to complete. Do not choose answers that contain responsibilities not requiring a nurse.**

EXAMPLE QUESTION:

A client who is 1-day postoperative for a cesarean section is to have her vital signs assessed, her abdominal dressing removed, assisted into the shower, and ambulated in the hallway with assistance. Which task should the nurse take responsibility for completing?

1. Assessing vital signs.
2. Removing the abdominal dressing.
3. Helping the client into the shower.
4. Walking the client in the hallway.

Answer: 1

Rationale: An unlicensed worker can easily complete answers 2, 3, and 4. A nurse should complete assessment of vital signs.

STRATEGY

> **Clients who have bilateral symptoms are usually not at risk. It is fairly common knowledge in the health care arena that when changes occur unilaterally, there is need for concern. Symmetry is seldom worrisome.**

EXAMPLE QUESTION:

A client comes to the clinic complaining of bilateral knee pain. He states that he was hiking this past weekend in the mountains on rough ground. He is worried because he had a cousin who died from bone cancer recently. He is requesting a full orthopedic workup. What is the *best response* for the nurse to make?

1. Assure the client that he does not have bone cancer.
2. Send the client for a full body magnetic resonance image immediately.
3. Obtain a sample of the client's blood for genetic testing.
4. Reassure the client that the doctor will see him and order testing if necessary.

Answer: 4

Rationale: Answer 1 has the nurse giving false reassurance. Answers 2 and 3 support the client's unrealistic fear that he has bone cancer. Answer 4 supports the theory that bilateral changes are not typically worrisome, and addresses the client's need to see his physician for assessment.

STRATEGY

Never choose answers that demonstrate the nurse completing a task "briskly." Remember, nurses perform most actions in moderation.

EXAMPLE QUESTION:

An elderly client is at risk of skin breakdown. The nurse knows that all the following interventions are useful in maintaining skin integrity *except*

1. Turning the client every 2 hours.
2. Massaging bony prominences briskly to stimulate circulation.
3. Providing the client with a diet high in protein.
4. Assessing the skin every shift.

Answer: 2

Rationale: Nurses do not perform actions "briskly." Nurses especially do not massage bony prominences. Answers 1, 3, and 4 are acceptable interventions in preventing skin breakdown.

STRATEGY

Avoid answers that encourage the use of hot and cold liquids. Nurses provide warm or cool liquids to prevent injury to the client.

EXAMPLE QUESTION:

A client is admitted with a diagnosis of deep vein thrombosis. The physician has ordered moist soaks with an aquapad to the affected extremity. The nurse would safely set the aquapad to which temperature setting?

1. Warm.
2. Hot.
3. Cool.
4. Cold.

Answer: 1

Rationale: Aquapads are for warm moist soaks. A temperature setting of hot would place the client at risk for burns. Cold and cool soaks are not used to treat deep vein thrombosis.

> **STRATEGY**
>
> **When teaching questions are confusing, you are unsure of what a question is asking, or a particular diagnosis is unfamiliar to you, choose the answer that you would consider best for the client in general.**

EXAMPLE QUESTION:

A mother of a 6-month-old infant newly diagnosed with intussusception comes to see the nurse. She has many questions regarding her infant's diagnosis, prognosis, and treatment plan. The nurse can best support the mother by making which of the following statements?

1. "Let me answer your questions one at a time."
2. "I will call the pediatrician's office now and set up an appointment for you to meet with him as soon as possible."

3. "It is impossible for me to know what the outcome of your baby's treatment will be."

4. "You need to be educated on the disease process, treatment options, and typical prognoses before I can answer your questions."

Answer: 1

Rationale: Answer 1 shows the mother you care, you are interested, and you are willing to help her. Answers 2, 3, and 4 do not foster communication or support the mother.

STRATEGY

Always look for clues in the stem of the question and try to match them with the points highlighted in the answers. Very often the same words will be present in the question as in the correct answer. Look for these similarities.

EXAMPLE QUESTION:

There are many government agencies with which health care workers should be familiar. One agency in particular is responsible for overseeing the enforcement of guidelines for workplace **safety** programs. That agency is known as the

1. Centers for Disease Control and Prevention.
2. U.S. Food and Drug Administration.
3. U.S. Department of Public Health.
4. Occupational **Safety** and Health Administration.

Answer: 4

Rationale: The word *safety* appears in the stem and in the answer.

In summary,

- Go with your instincts when you apply these skills and strategies! When knowledge and intuition are applied using the tools presented in this text, it is a winning combination.
- A student once told me she has many "inner monologues." I encourage you to have these internal discussions as you learn and apply the tools offered here. It is a wonderful way to reinforce what you have learned and is useful for recall of information.

USING A MNEMONIC SYSTEM

Using a mnemonic system to assist in answering questions correctly is strongly suggested. A mnemonic is a word or phrase that helps you to associate facts and information. This association is useful in supplementing a test-takers memory. Examples of mnemonic tactics are as follows:

STRATEGY

When referring to fetal heart rate decelerations, remember the following associations: *early* decelerations are caused by fetal h*ead* compression. Look for the letters "EA" in E*A*rly and h*EA*d. *La*te decelerations are caused by p*la*cental insufficiency. Look for the "LA" in L*A*te and p*LA*centa. *Variable* decelerations are associated with *u*mbilical cord compression. Look for the "U" and "V," both of which come at the end of the alphabet.

STRATEGY

When placing cardiac electrodes on the chest of a client, remember to place the *white* electrode on the *right* side of the chest (note the rhyme) and place the *black* (representative of smoke) above the heart on the left and the *red* (representative of fire) below the heart, remembering that smoke comes before, or rises above, fire.

When examining a pregnant woman for signs and symptoms of pregnancy, remember the alphabet ABCDEF*GH*. Chadwick's sign reflects vaginal changes, *Goodell's* sign reflects cervical changes, and *Hagar's* sign reflects lower uterine segment changes. Anatomically, the vagina is seen before the cervix, and the lower uterine segment is visualized after the cervix. Hence, remembering that *C* comes before *G*, which comes before *H*, helps the test-taker to remember what changes apply to these reproductive structures.

When instilling eardrops in the child and the adult, remember to pull the lobe *up* and back for the ad*u*lt and *down* and back for the chil*d*. Note the "U" in Up and adUlt and the "D" in Down and chilD. Also, you can remember that up is to tall as down is to small. In other words, a tall adult and a small child.

For the client with congestive heart failure, left-sided failure causes pulmonary edema or edema of the lungs. Right-sided failure causes peripheral edema. Note the "L" in Left and Lungs. If you learn to associate *l*eft-sided failure with the *l*ungs, right-sided failure also becomes easier to remember.

Remembering the antidote for commonly administered medications is easier when associative cues are used. For example, the antidote for *H*eparin is *P*rotamine sulfate. Note the "H" and "P," as in *H*ewlett-*P*ackard, the well-known computer, printer, and camera products company. The antidote for *C*oumadin is vitamin *K*. Note the "C" and "K," as in Calvin *K*lein, a well-known clothing manufacturer and fashion designer.

STRATEGY

Recalling the treatment protocol for clients with sickle cell disease can be associated with *HHOP*. *H*eat, *h*ydration, *o*xygen, and *p*ain medications are priority interventions for the client in a crisis.

STRATEGY

When remembering the blood vessels found in a fetal/newborn umbilical cord, you can name the cord AVA, which stands for Artery, Vein, Artery.

SUMMARY

One of the most important skill and strategy a test-taker can remember is to approach any examination in a state of preparedness. By this I mean well studied, knowledgeable, and confident and, perhaps equally essential to the testing process, managing a low to moderate level of anxiety. Some degree of anxiety will help you to strive to do your best. Anxiety can be a powerful motivator, but high levels of anxiety can cause you to experience physical and emotional exhaustion. When you reach this level of apprehension, a testing situation quickly becomes a nightmare and your mind will flood with worry and doubt. So do yourself a favor and keep reading. By the time you reach Chapter 6 you will be equipped with all the tools, skills, and strategies to go to your testing situation in the best possible intellectual, physical, and emotional condition as possible. Now—go for it!

START WITH THE BASICS

Beginning the process of answering NCLEX questions correctly starts with accurately reading the question. This sounds too basic, I know. But I have found over the years that many questions, if not most, are answered incorrectly because the test-taker simply did not read the question carefully enough to really understand what the question is asking.

STRATEGY

I recommend that it is best to *read each question twice*: the first time to generally get an idea about what the question is asking and the second time to intently concentrate on what is being referenced.

This may sound time consuming, and it can be without practice. Any tactic that is practiced over and over again eventually comes to you naturally and with greater speed. The same is true when practicing test-taking skills and strategies. The more often the behavior is performed, the more proficient the test-taker becomes at mastering the technique.

After the question is read for the second time, have what I call an "inner monologue" with yourself. Talk to your own mind and ask yourself, "Do I truly understand what the question is asking?" Once you believe you have a clear perception of the question, pick out what are defined as "**key**" words.

STRATEGY

Key words are found in the stem of the question and function as guides to the correct answer.

These words are *intentionally* used by item writers and should be heavily considered when selecting an answer. Examples of these key words include the following:

- First
- Most
- Least
- Best
- Priority
- Initial
- Contraindicated
- Avoid
- Except
- Never
- All
- Always
- Only
- Assessment
- Plan/goal
- Intervention/action
- Evaluation

Very often these words are *italicized*, written in **bold**, and/or <u>underlined</u>. This is to call attention to them. Do not ignore these words. They typically reflect the guiding principles item writers frequently follow when creating NCLEX questions. Examples of these principles include the following:

> **Key words reflect the guiding principles item writers follow.**

- Safety for the client is paramount.
- Choose the answer that is the priority assessment or action for the nurse.
- Select the answer that reflects a life-threatening situation for the client.

- Nurses **A**ssess **B**efore **C**aring.
- Remember **A**irway, **B**reathing, and **C**irculation.
- It is generally acceptable to address the physiological concerns of the client before addressing his or her psychological needs.
- It is routinely appropriate to consider the first sign and symptom mentioned in the question as the most important.

Once you have read the question twice, asked yourself what the question is really asking, picked out the key words, and believe you are ready to proceed, you are then prepared to apply the 5-Step Approach. Again, if this all seems too time consuming, let me assure you that practice makes this process short and concise. It is imperative that every aspect of the process is carried out with each question. Repetition, repetition, repetition is fundamental to mastering the approach.

Repetition, repetition, repetition.

Once this is done, you are ready to read each answer one time *without* selecting the correct answer. Then re-read the answers and apply the 5-Step Approach as described below.

THE 5-STEP APPROACH

Step 1

STRATEGY

After reading each answer twice, rate each answer on a scale of 1 to 5, with 5 as the *best* possible answer and 1 as the *worst* possible answer.

Assign each answer a number in an orderly manner. In other words, rate each answer in the order they appear. Do not skip around from one answer to another. Use number 3 when you are not sure of an answer or if you have no idea if an answer is right or wrong. I call this the "middle of the road number." If step 1 is used correctly, you will answer 95% of all questions without going any further. Once this is done, choose the answer that has the highest number. You may use each number more than once. Do not concern yourself at this point if two answers have the same high number. How to deal with this situation is also covered.

EXAMPLE QUESTION:

A postoperative client has been put on a clear liquid diet. Which item may be ordered by the nurse as an appropriate mid-afternoon snack?

1. A vanilla milkshake.
2. A plain yogurt.
3. A glass of apple juice.
4. A small container of milk.

Answer: 3

Rationale: Answers 1, 2, and 4 are items listed on a full liquid diet and therefore should be rated as a "1" or a "2." Answer 3 is an item usually included on a clear liquid diet and therefore should be rated as a "4" or a "5."

Client Need: Health Promotion and Maintenance

It is possible to have the same number for more than one answer. When this occurs, you should still choose the answer with the highest number rating. It is then time to move on to the next question.

EXAMPLE QUESTION:

A client is admitted with a diagnosis of acute gastroenteritis. The nurse anticipates meeting the client's nutritional needs by administering the following:

1. A full liquid diet.
2. A clear liquid diet.
3. Intravenous fluids.
4. Food and liquids as tolerated.

Answer: 3

Rationale: The client with acute gastroenteritis is usually placed on NPO with intravenous hydration. Answers 1 and 2 might both receive a "3" rating if the reader is unsure or a "2" rating if the test-taker is fairly confident they are incorrect. With both answers having the same low rating, the reader would eliminate them. Answer 4 should be eliminated and rated as "1." Answer 3 is correct and should be rated as "4" or "5."

Client Need: Physiological Integrity

If you have more than one answer with the same high number or are not sure of any of the distracters, you must then go to step 2 of the 5-Step Approach.

EXAMPLE QUESTION:

A client on postoperative day 2 complains of incisional pain. Which action would be a priority for the nurse?

1. Determine the time the last dose of pain medication was administered.
2. Assess the client's vital signs, including temperature.
3. Have the client describe the pain and rate it on a scale of 1 to10.
4. Provide comfort measures such as repositioning and a back rub.

Answer: 3

Rationale: It may be easy for the test-taker to be confused between answers 1 and 3 because they both refer to the client's physiological integrity. Scoring them both with a high number, such as a "5," may further confuse the test-taker. It is important to keep in mind that the nurse must assess the pain first to initially determine if pain medication is appropriate. Remember, nurses **A**ssess **B**efore **C**aring!

Client Need: Physiological Integrity

Step 2

STRATEGY

> **If step 1 has not led you to the right answer, use step 2. In this step choose the answer that reflects the Client Need referenced in the question.**

If the question refers to the Physiological Integrity of the client, choose the corresponding answer that contains the same physiological need of the client. The same is true for psychological integrity, and the other client needs.

EXAMPLE QUESTION:

A client is admitted to your psychiatric unit with a diagnosis of anxiety, panic-level. After showing the client to his room, what initial action by the nurse would be most therapeutic?

1. Place the client in bed with the side rails up.
2. Remain with the client.
3. Medicate the client with a sedative.
4. Have the client join a unit exercise group immediately.

Answer: 2

Rationale: A client experiencing panic-level anxiety should not be left alone. Answers 1, 3, and 4 address Physiological Integrity of the client. Answer 2 addresses the Psychosocial Integrity of the client, as referenced in the question.

Client Need: Psychosocial Integrity

After choosing the correct answer, move onto the next question. If more than one answer contains the Client Need referenced in the question and a priority cannot be determined, you must move to the next step.

Step 3

If step 2 does not assist you in finding the correct answer to the question, use step 3. Step 3 directs the test-taker to choose the answer that reflects the Integrated Process referenced in the question.

If the question speaks to Communication and Documentation, choose the corresponding answer that discusses how nurses communicate with clients and document assessments and care. The same is true for Teaching and Learning, and the other integrated processes.

EXAMPLE QUESTION:

The nurse is assessing the newly admitted client. The client is scheduled for exploratory abdominal surgery in 2 hours. The nurse completes an admission assessment and discovers the client has mild anxiety regarding the surgery, last had food and fluids at 11:30 p.m. the night before, and signed the surgical consent at the doctor's office 2 days ago. What would be the nurse's next intervention?

1. Call the anesthesiologist to sedate the client.
2. Notify the surgeon of the client's food and fluid consumption.
3. Witness the surgical consent.
4. Document the findings on the client's chart.

Answer: 4

Rationale: All the assessment data are normal and should be *documented* on the client's chart. There is no need to sedate the client. It is appropriate that the client has been NPO since midnight, and the nurse cannot witness the surgical consent because the nurse was not present when the consent was signed.

Integrated Process: Communication and Documentation

After choosing the correct answer, go on to the next question. If more than one distracter suggests communication and documentation and a priority action is undeterminable, you must move to the next step.

Step 4

If step 3 does not yield a single answer, go to step 4. Here you are to choose the answer that stands alone.

There are two ways to decide that an answer stands alone. First, look for the one answer that contains content dissimilar to the other three answers. The dissimilarity may indicate the answer is correct.

EXAMPLE QUESTION:

A client is ordered on a low sodium diet. The client's family has requested to bring in some favorite foods. What food item should the nurse tell the family members to omit?

1.   Boiled rice.
2.   Flat bread.
3.   Broiled fish fillet.
4.   Pickled vegetables.

Answer: 4

Rationale: Answers 1, 2, and 3 are naturally low in sodium. Answer 4 has a high sodium content. Therefore answer 4 stands alone.

Client Need: Physiological Integrity

Second, look for the one answer that is noticeably shorter or longer than the three remaining answers. Occasionally, the shortest or the longest answers should be considered correct. If you decide to select the longest answer, remember this tactic is related to the strategy that directs you to choose the answer that is the most comprehensive.

EXAMPLE QUESTION:

A client is to have an abdominal paracentesis. The nurse knows the position of choice for this procedure is

1. Prone.
2. Supine.
3. Lateral.
4. Sitting up with feet supported.

Answer: 4

Rationale: Answer 4 stands alone in that it is the longest answer. Answers 1, 2, and 3 are the shortest and are incorrect.

Client Need: Physiological Integrity

After opting for the answer that stands alone, move onto the next question. If there is not a single answer standing by itself, go to step 5.

Step 5

STRATEGY

If step 4 does not lead you to a satisfactory answer, use step 5. Step 5 is simply choosing answer "C" or "3," because statistical research shows that over 30% of all multiple choice answers are "C" or "3."

This step, when *used appropriately and not abused*, will work and improve your guessing ability dramatically.

EXAMPLE QUESTION:

A client is selecting foods for the next day's meals. Which meal selection would the nurse consider to be nutritionally superior?

1. Ham, cheese, and mustard on rye bread, gelatin, and apple juice.
2. Broiled lamb chop, peas, French fried potatoes, and black coffee.
3. Baked chicken, white rice, broccoli, and skim milk.
4. A three-egg omelet, lean bacon, orange juice, and white toast.

Answer: 3

Rationale: Chicken is high in protein and low in fat. White rice and broccoli are high in vitamins and minerals. Ham, French fried potatoes, and lean bacon are high in sodium and fat. If the answer is not clear, use step 5 and choose answer "C" or "3."

Client Need: Physiological Integrity

Random guessing results in approximately a 25% success rate. Using step 5 wisely and *only when steps 1 through 4 have been exhausted* increases your success at guessing to greater than 35%. This is the hardest step for test-takers to trust and to use *judiciously*. Remember, application of this step helps you only when you have gone through steps 1 through 4 and have not been able to answer the question.

ALTERNATIVES TO NUMBERING ANSWERS OR USING STEP 1

There are complementary methods for answering teaching questions. By this I mean questions that ask the test-taker to determine when teaching has been effective or to determine when more teaching is needed. This method is to assign Bs for "bad" answers and Gs for "good" answers.

STRATEGY

If a question asks the nurse to determine that teaching was effective, you would assign three Bs and one G. In other words, three answers have bad information and one answer has good information.

The good information is the correct answer. Hence, you will determine the single statement that tells the nurse that teaching was understood.

EXAMPLE QUESTION:

The nurse is teaching a preoperative client how to do deep breathing exercises and cough effectively after surgery. Which statement made by the client would indicate to the nurse that teaching has been effective?

1. "I will splint my incision with a pillow to cough."
2. "I will ask for pain medication only after my deep breathing exercises."
3. "I will avoid using the incentive spirometer until I can get out of bed alone."
4. "I will deep breathe and cough every 4 hours."

Answer: 1

Rationale: Answers 2, 3, and 4 are clearly bad things for a client to say. Pain medication should be given beforehand, the incentive spirometer should be used while the client is on bed rest or is immobile, and deep breathing and coughing should be done every hour. Hence, answers 2, 3, and 4 would be labeled with a "B" and answer 1 would be labeled with a "G."

> **Did you notice that answer #2 had the key word "only" and should be automatically eliminated?**

Client Need: Physiological Integrity

STRATEGY **If a question asks the nurse to decide that teaching was not effective, you would assign three Gs and one B. In other words you will have three answers that are good things and one answer that is a bad thing.**

The answer with bad information is the correct answer. If done this way, you will reach the single answer that tells the nurse that his or her teaching was *not* understood.

EXAMPLE QUESTION:

A nurse is teaching a preoperative client how to do deep breathing exercises and cough effectively after surgery. Which statement made by the client would indicate to the nurse that additional teaching is needed?

1. "I will splint my incision with a pillow to cough."
2. "I will ask for pain medication before doing my deep breathing exercises."
3. "I will continue using the incentive spirometer until I can ambulate alone."
4. "I will deep breathe and cough every 4 hours."

Answer: 4

Rationale: Answers 1, 2, and 3 are all correct statements and would be assigned a "G." Answer 4 is an incorrect statement because the client must deep breath and cough more frequently and therefore would be assigned a "B."

Client Need: Physiological Integrity

If a question asks the test-taker to determine a fact, I recommend labeling the answer with a "T" for true or an "F" for false. The "fact" answer would be labeled with a "T" and the other three distracters that do not answer the question would be labeled with "Fs."

EXAMPLE QUESTION:

What is the most important step a nurse can take to prevent the spread of infection?

1. Wash your hands frequently.
2. Change your gloves often.
3. Apply asepsis for dressing changes.
4. Change bed linens daily.

Answer: 1

Rationale: Answer 1 is a fact. Hand washing has proven to be the best preventive measure in stopping the spread of infection. Changing gloves often, using asepsis for dressing changes, and changing bed linens have not proven to stop the spread of infection to any great degree. Gloves should be changed after each use, sterile technique is used for dressing changes, and bed linen should be changed as necessary. Hence, answer 1 would be labeled with a "T" and answers 2, 3, and 4 would be labeled with an "F."

Client Need: Safe, Effective Care Environment

PRACTICE AND HABITS

It is common knowledge that, as humans, we have habits. Some are noticeable and others are not. You may want to ask yourself what habits you have. And then, how these habits became a part of your activities of daily living.

Also, ask yourself what specific habits you possess regarding test-taking. Habits become a part of our lives as we perform them repeatedly, or practice if you will, because they give us feelings of comfort and security, and we most often repeatedly do so unconsciously.

STRATEGY

> **With daily repetition, applying the approach you have just learned will become your new test-taking habit and replace the habits you have now for taking a test.**

Application of the 5-Step Approach, if skillfully rehearsed, will become your new test-taking habit. But do not fool yourself. Taking the NCLEX is a stressful event, and if using the 5-Step Approach has not truly become a natural habit, when faced with the stress of the examination you will likely turn to your old test-taking habits for support.

Make a promise to yourself now that you will not answer another test question without using the 5-Step Approach, regardless of the level of difficulty or your degree of confidence in an answer. As I tell my students after each review course, once the NCLEX is behind you, use whatever test-taking skills and strategies you want but until then trust in the approach and make it a part of your daily activities of living. Well done!

PRACTICE QUESTIONS

A nurse is to administer an intermittent tube feeding through a nasogastric tube for the client. The nurse is to check for gastric residual before administering the feeding. The nurse understands that the rationale for checking gastric residual before administering any tube feeding is to

1. Confirm that the nasogastric tube is properly placed.
2. Assess for the digestion of the previous tube feeding formula.
3. Assess the status of the client's fluid and electrolyte balance.
4. Assess how much of the last feeding was absorbed.

Answer: 4

Rationale: It is imperative that the nurse assess the amount of unabsorbed feeding from the previous administration. This assists the nurse to not overfeed the client and to not cause distention of the stomach.

Client Need: Physiological Integrity

A client is admitted to a psychiatric unit with a diagnosis of major depression. The nurse completes an admission assessment on the client and determines that he is suffering from poor nutritional intake. A diagnosis of altered nutrition is made. A priority nursing action related to this concern is

1. Educate the client regarding the importance of eating good nutritional food.
2. Weigh the client every morning and document findings on the client's chart.
3. Inform the client's psychiatrist of your nutritional concern for this client, and ask him to order a nutritional consultation.
4. Contact the nutritionist, offer the client frequent small meals every few hours, and schedule time to sit with the client during these meals.

Answer: 4

Rationale: A change in appetite is a major symptom of depression. Offering the client frequent small meals and being present during that time to support and encourage the client is an appropriate nursing intervention. A depressed client is not open to learning about nutrition. Weighing the client does nothing to assist in increasing nutritional intake. Also, answer 4 is the most comprehensive answer with all accurate information.

Client Need: Physiological Integrity

A nursing instructor is questioning a nursing student regarding the cause of hemophilia. The nursing student correctly responds by telling the instructor that (select all that apply)

1. Hemophilia is an X-linked hereditary disorder.
2. Sons inherit hemophilia from their fathers.
3. Daughters inherit hemophilia from their mothers.
4. Hemophilia A results from a deficiency of factor VIII.
5. Hemophilia B results from a deficiency of factor IX.
6. Sons inherit hemophilia from their mothers.

Answer: 1, 4, 5, and 6

Rationale: Hemophilia is an X-linked hereditary disorder. Sons inherit hemophilia from their mothers, and daughters inherit the carrier status from their fathers. Hemophilia A results from a deficiency of factor XIII, and hemophilia B results from a deficiency of factor IX.

Client Need: Physiological Integrity

A child is admitted to the pediatric unit with a diagnosis of a brain tumor. The nurse is responsible for ensuring a safe health care environment for this child. Which of the following should the nurse include as a *priority* action in the plan of care for this pediatric client?

1. Do not allow the child to ambulate in his room alone.
2. Do not allow the child to come in contact with other pediatric clients.
3. Initiate seizure precautions.
4. Have the child use a wheelchair for all out of bed activities.

Answer: 3

Rationale: Seizure precautions for all pediatric clients with a diagnosis of brain tumor are a priority for the nurse. Safety is the priority. Options

1, 2, and 4 are not necessary to keep the client safe, unless ordered by the physician.

Client Need: Safe, Effective Care Environment

A pregnant client at 37 weeks is admitted to the labor and delivery unit. A nurse is assisting in caring for this client and notes a diagnosis of placenta previa. The labor and delivery nurse knows that an internal cervical examination will *not* be performed on this client primarily because it could

1. Introduce infection.
2. Initiate preterm labor.
3. Cause profound bleeding.
4. Rupture the fetal membranes.

Answer: 3

Rationale: When placenta previa is suspected or known, cervical exams are not performed. This is because any pressure applied to the placenta could cause a premature separation of the placenta and heavy bleeding. Remember: airway, breathing, and **circulation**. The priority here is preventing hemorrhage. Infection is a risk with multiple internal exams.

Client Need: Physiological Integrity

A new mother is breastfeeding her newborn infant. The mother complains to the nurse that her nipples are sore. The nurse provides which of the following suggestions to the client in assisting in the healing of sore nipples?

1. Avoid rotating breastfeeding positions so that the nipples toughen.
2. Stop breastfeeding when the nipples are sore to allow time to heal.
3. Have the mother nurse less frequently and offer a bottle in between nursing until the nipples are less sore.
4. Change the position of the newborn infant on the nipples with each feeding.

Answer: 4

Rationale: Changing the position of the newborn on the nipples with each feeding helps to reduce soreness. Options 1, 2, and 3 do not help in reducing soreness of nipples and contain incorrect information.

Client Need: Health Promotion and Maintenance

....

A nurse sees a nursing assistant preparing to deliver a food tray to an Orthodox Jewish client. The nurse observes the food on the tray and notes that there is a roast beef dinner with skim milk. Which action should the nurse tell the nursing assistant to take?

1. Have the assistant deliver the food tray to the client.
2. Call the dietary department and ask for a different tray.
3. Replace the skim milk with low-fat cream.
4. Asked the dietary department to send up a chicken dinner to replace the roast beef.

Answer: 2

Rationale: A meal with dairy–meat combination is not acceptable in the Orthodox Jewish tradition. The nurse would not deliver the tray or change any of the items. A new tray should be obtained from the dietary department.

Client Need: Psychosocial Integrity

WHAT ARE ALTERNATE FORMAT QUESTIONS?

For years the NCLEX consisted of standard multiple choice questions. This involved a question, known as the stem, and one correct answer and three or more wrong answers, known as distracters. A distracter's purpose is to divert the test-taker's attention away from the correct answer. The test-taker was asked to eliminate all but one option and respond to the question with the remaining answer. It was commonly thought that two of the four answers could be easily eliminated, leaving the test-taker struggling with the remaining two. This has changed over time as item writers for the NCLEX, as with nursing faculty across the country, are attempting to write questions that have four correct answers, with one option as the *priority*.

In recent years the National Council of State Boards of Nursing has designed alternate format questions as adjunctive testing of nursing knowledge. Although most test questions on the NCLEX remain standard multiple choice questions, 5% to 10% of the questions are alternate format questions. It is thought that the rationale for this change was to test the critical thinking abilities of the nurses seeking licensure. The types of alternate format questions to be discussed include the following:

- Multiple response multiple choice questions
- Prioritizing/ordering response questions
- Fill in the blank questions
- Image/hot spot questions

Multiple Response Multiple Choice Questions

STRATEGY

Multiple response multiple choice questions consist of a stem and four or more (usually a minimum of five) options. The test-taker must read the question and choose one or more answers, or *all that apply.*

This includes the best possible answers and all related responses. When a correct answer is omitted by the test-taker or when an incorrect answer is included by the test-taker, the entire question is marked as wrong. *There is no partial credit given on the NCLEX.* It is strongly suggested that at least two responses be chosen. There have been multiple response multiple choice questions in NCLEX review books where there was only one correct answer, and there have been questions where all of the options were correct, but these examples are rarely seen. There is no way to determine how many options are applicable. Each multiple response multiple choice question is to be addressed separately.

EXAMPLE QUESTION:

A 20-year-old female client is admitted with an eating disorder and has a nursing diagnosis of Altered Nutrition: Less Than Body Requirements. Which of the following nursing interventions would be **best** for this client? Select all that apply.

1. Provide the client with small frequent meals.
2. Monitor weight daily.
3. Allow the client to choose the meals she will eat.
4. Encourage the client to express her feelings.
5. Stay with the client during mealtime and for 1 hour afterward.
6. Insist the client eat three substantial meals each day.

Answers: 1, 2, 4, and 5

Rationale: Smaller meals are usually tolerated well by most clients. Monitoring weight daily does not allow the client to hide weight loss. Expressing feelings can be very therapeutic. Staying with the client allows the nurse to accurately document total intake and prevents the client from purging after eating. Allowing the client to choose what meals she will eat will foster the client's desire to skip eating. Nurses are not therapeutic when "insisting" a client comply, nor do they promote "substantial" or large meals. Remember these strategies?

Client Need: Psychosocial Integrity

Prioritizing/Ordering Response Questions

STRATEGY

A prioritizing/ordering response question contains all correct answers. In other words, the nurse is to complete all the assessments listed or perform all the interventions included in the answer section of the question. The test-taker is asked to prioritize the responses in the order in which they are to be performed.

Here the test-taker is being judged on his or her ability to determine the order in which tasks are to be completed. A numbering system is used, with 1 assigned to the first, or most important, task to be completed, 2 assigned to the second most important task to be completed, and so on. The highest number is assigned to the task to be completed last. If any number in the sequencing is out of order, the entire question is marked wrong. Numbers are used only **once**.

EXAMPLE QUESTION:

A client is to receive 1 unit of packed red blood cells. The nurse responsible for administering the blood will complete all the following assessments and interventions. Number the nurse's actions in the order they are to be performed.

_____ Assess the client's vital signs.
_____ Start an intravenous solution of normal saline.
_____ Return the used blood bag to the blood bank.
_____ Remain with the client for the first 15 minutes of the transfusion.
_____ Reassess the client's vital signs.

Answers: 2, 1, 5, 3, and 4

Rationale: The nurse would first start an intravenous infusion of normal saline. The nurse would then assess the client's vital signs before hanging the blood. The client should not be left unattended for the first 15 minutes of the transfusion because of the risk of an allergic reaction. After that time, the vitals are reassessed. Finally, when the transfusion is finished, the used blood bag is returned to the blood bank.

Client Need: Safe, Effective Care Environment

Fill-in-the-Blank Questions

STRATEGY

The answers for fill-in-the-blank questions are to be provided by the test-taker.

There is not a list to choose from, so the test-taker is asked to enter the necessary information on a line located after the question. Spelling is a factor. The computer must be able to recognize the word or phrase typed on the option line as the exact answer required. Also, many fill-in-the-blank questions are mathematical calculations, either dosage calculations or intravenous administration. It is important to remember that you should give only the information asked for in the stem. Do not embellish your answers. If the question asks for the number of milliliters to be given, write the number only, not the number and the label "ml." In other words, all mathematical answers have labels, such as ml, gtts/min, ml/hr, tablets, units, and so on. If the stem contains the label as part of the question, provide the numerical part of the answer only. If the stem does not contain the label as part of the question, you *must* include the label in your answer or the response will be marked wrong.

EXAMPLE QUESTION:

A nurse is assessing a newborn on delivery day 2. The nurse notes a raised bruised area on the left side of the neonate's scalp that does not cross the suture line. The nurse would correctly document this finding as a(n)

Answer: Cephalhematoma

Rationale: A cephalhematoma is a swelling of the subcutaneous tissue of the newborn's scalp with blood. The collection of blood is located beneath the periosteum of the cranial bone and therefore does not cross the suture line.

Client Need: Physiological Integrity

EXAMPLE QUESTION:

A nurse is assigned to administer 1000 ml of dextrose 5% water to her or his client every 8 hours. The drop factor on the tubing is 10 gtts/ml. The nurse would correctly set the infusion pump to run at *how many ml per hour*?

Answer: 125

Rationale: 1000 ml divided by 8 hours equals 125 ml/hour. The label "ml" is not included in the answer because the question asks how many ml per hour to set the pump.

Client Need: Safe, Effective Care Environment

Image/Hot Spot Questions

In image/hot spot questions, the NCLEX provides the test-taker with a picture or drawing and asks you to do one of two things. The first task you may be asked to perform is to identify what the illustration is portraying, what is wrong with the illustration, or what part of the illustration is referenced in the question. You may have to choose from a multiple choice list or type your response on an option line to answer this question. The second kind of image/hot spot question is one that asks the test-taker to mark the correct area on a graphic design.

The test-taker is asked to move the cursor over the correct position of the graphic design and mark the area with an "X." To help the test-taker, as the cursor is moved over the illustration, boxes occasionally open. The test-taker should choose the box nearest the correct area to place the "X" and answer the question. It is important to be as precise as possible when selecting the site for placement of the "X."

EXAMPLE QUESTION:

Below is a representation of the female reproductive organs. What number on the diagram represents the most commonly assessed organ(s) for ectopic pregnancy?

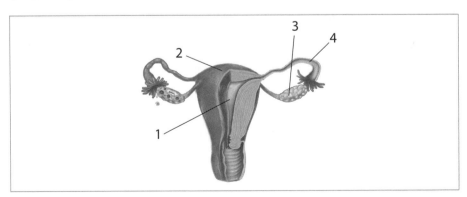

Answer: 4

Rationale: An ectopic pregnancy is when a fertilized ovum implants outside of the uterine cavity. The fallopian tubes are the most common location for ectopic pregnancy, accounting for 95% of all extrauterine pregnancies.

Client Need: Physiological Integrity

EXAMPLE QUESTION:

A client in rehabilitation is recovering from a mild stroke. The client is experiencing difficulties with his balance. The nurse identifies the area of the brain that controls this function on the graphic below. Mark the correct area with an "X."

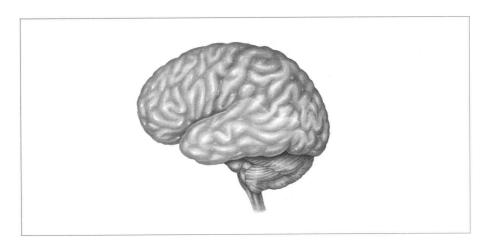

Answer: The cerebellum

Rationale: The cerebellum is the area of the brain that controls balance and other motor functions.

Client Need: Physiological Integrity

SUMMARY

There is no doubt that there are challenges for the test-taker to overcome when answering alternate format questions. These challenges include scrutinizing the test-takers ability to

- Prioritize
- Render complete care
- Assess/intervene competently
- Problem solve
- Spell
- Orchestrate step by step nursing care in a clinical scenario
- Critically think
- Calculate
- Maintain client safety
- Eliminate irrelevant information and options

PRACTICE QUESTIONS

A nurse is caring for a client who is postoperative. The client has had a cholecystectomy and is complaining of pain. Which of the following actions should the nurse take? Select all that apply.

1. Offer the client a back rub.
2. Medicate the client with the prescribed analgesic.
3. Assess the client's pain level on a scale from 1 to 10.
4. Notify the surgeon.
5. Change the client's position.

Answers: 1, 2, 3, and 5

Rationale: Nonpharmacologic remedies are often helpful is diminishing a client's pain. Properly assessing the pain and giving appropriate medication are important. There is no indication that the surgeon needs to be notified.

Client Need: Physiological Integrity

An 85-year-old client has just had surgery. The physician orders Demerol (meperidine hydrochloride) 30 mg intramuscularly every 4 hours as needed. The label on the syringe reads 50 mg per 3 ml. How many milliliters should the nurse discard?

Answer: 1.2

Rationale: The doctor ordered 30 mg. When 30 mg is divided by 50 mg × 3 ml, the answer is 1.8 ml. This is the amount to administer. When 1.8 is subtracted from 3, the remainder is 1.2. The amount of medication to be discarded is 1.2 ml.

Client Need: Physiological Integrity

A cardiac client is to receive Lasix (furosemide) 40 mg by mouth. The nurse notes that the client has not been receiving supplemental electrolytes. Which laboratory value would be a *priority* for the nurse to assess before administering the Lasix?

Answer: Potassium

Rationale: Lasix is a loop diuretic and therefore promotes excretion of potassium. The nurse should monitor the client's serum potassium level before administering the Lasix to prevent hypokalemia.

Client Need: Physiological Integrity

A nurse is caring for an elderly client who just underwent a cardiac catheterization. Which *priority* nursing interventions should be included in the client's plan of care for the next 8 hours? Select all that apply.

1. Maintain pressure over the femoral puncture site.
2. Place the client in high Fowler's position.
3. Assess the femoral dressing for drainage and bleeding.
4. Monitor the client's vital signs every 4 hours and document.
5. Keep the client's hip and leg extended.
6. Allow the client bathroom privileges.

Answers: 1, 3, and 5

Rationale: Maintaining pressure over the puncture site prevents bleeding and promotes clot formation. Vital signs should be assessed every 15 minutes for the first hour and every 30 minutes for the second hour. Vital signs should then be assessed every hour for the next 4 hours. Assessing the dressing frequently alerts the nurse to bleeding. Preventing the leg and hip from flexing also helps to promote clot formation. Preventing bleeding is the priority safety issue.

Client Need: Physiological Integrity

A client comes to the clinic after insertion of a permanent pacemaker for postoperative assessment. Which of the following instructions should the nurse include in the client's teaching plan? Select all that apply.

1. Count the heart rate for 1 minute each morning.
2. Count the respiratory rate for 1 minute each morning.
3. Call the clinic if there is redness or swelling at the insertion site.
4. Avoid coming into contact with metal detectors.
5. Avoid microwave ovens.

Answers: 1, 3, and 5

Rationale: A client with a permanent pacemaker should count their heart rate daily and record the information. The nurse should teach the importance of reporting a heart rate that is too slow or too fast. The nurse should also teach the client the signs and symptoms of potential infection at the insertion site. Microwave ovens have been known to disrupt the functioning of the pacemaker. Assessing the respiratory rate is not necessary, and metal detectors will not harm the pacemaker.

Client Need: Physiological Integrity

A client with angina comes to the emergency room. Which of the following signs and symptoms should the nurse expect the client to exhibit? Select all that apply.

1. Tightness in the chest.
2. General muscle cramping.
3. Pressure on the chest.
4. Jaw pain.
5. Bradypnea.
6. Bradycardia.

Answers: 1, 3, and 4

Rationale: A patent with angina frequently complains of tightness in the chest, chest pressure, and jaw pain. General muscle cramping is not associated with angina. Bradypnea and bradycardia are also not associated with angina.

Client Need: Physiological Integrity

The nurse is assessing the peripheral pulses of a newly admitted cardiac client. Identify the area where the nurse would palpate the left pedal pulse.

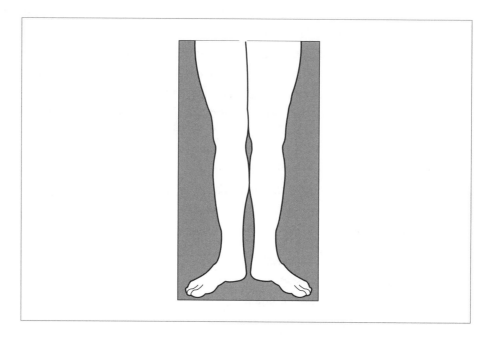

Answer: The "X" would appear on the top of the foot.

Rationale: The pedal pulse is located on the top of the foot.

Client Need: Physiological Integrity

A nursing home nurse enters the day room and finds the window curtains on fire. The nurse performs all the following actions. List the nursing actions in the priority order the nurse should complete them.

___ Close the door.
___ Sound the fire alarm.
___ Remove the residents from the room.
___ Document the nurse's observations.
___ Extinguish the fire.

Answers: 3, 2, 1, 5, and 4

Rationale: The nurse's priority action is to remove the residents from danger. The nurse would then sound the fire alarm and close the door to contain the fire. If able, the nurse would extinguish the fire. The last thing the nurse would do is to document the occurrence on an incident report. Remember the acronym "RACE": rescue, alarm, confine, and extinguish.

Client Need: Safe, Effective Care Environment

WHAT'S NEXT?

Now that you have prepared your intellectual mind for the NCLEX, it is time to prepare yourself physically and emotionally. There are ways to help yourself feel better physically and emotionally. Conditioning your body and mind to be successful is part of the preparatory directions I give to my students. It is a way to work on overcoming fear, specifically fear of the unknown. Fear of the unknown is an extremely strong emotion and, if not dealt with, can become overwhelming.

OVERCOMING FEAR

Once you receive the information concerning where and when you are going to test, it is advisable that you go to the testing site as soon as possible. Once you arrive, go inside the testing site and glance around. Next, speak to the receptionist, introduce yourself, and ask to see the testing area. Look all around, examine the computers, and visit the restrooms. I recommend that you familiarize yourself with the test area, both inside and outside the building. Take mental pictures and try to imagine yourself there, sitting at a computer and using the facilities. One of the biggest fears my students share with me is their fear of the unfamiliarity of the testing site. They wonder where they will be on the day of the test, what the computers look like, and where they will park. Making this trip

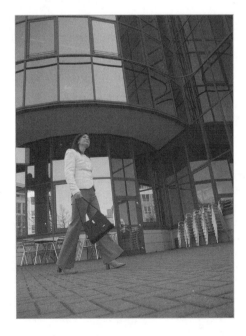

before the day of the examination eliminates one of the greatest fears associated
with testing, that is, wondering what it will
be like on the big day. Eliminating as much

> **Eliminate the fear of the unknown.**

fear as possible before you sit down to the test is an advantage for you.

TALK TO YOURSELF

Another helpful suggestion I offer my students is to talk to their subconscious minds by repeating positive affirmations. Speaking positive affirmations out loud is a widely used technique to build our self-esteem, to boost our self-concept, and to emotionally stabilize our feelings. I remember when my son was a young child. He wanted to ride a two-wheel bike more than anything, but for some reason he did not have the balance to stay upright. He would watch his friends ride their bikes and wish he could do the same. I decided to give him the same power of suggestion I give to my students before a test. I took him outside and I taught him to talk to himself by repeating positive affirmations. I had him talk to his bike, to tell his bike he was the master and he was in control. I had him repeat again and again that he was going to ride his bike because he was the boss! He said the words over and over. I stepped back and watched him transform from an upset little boy to a determined little man. Within minutes my son got on his bike and rode away. He was a little wobbly and used my neighbor's garage door to stop, but the point is he rode the bike. And he was thrilled. He yelled to me that he was the master of his bike! I had given my son a very powerful tool. Today he is 26 years old, a newlywed, and has a successful career. He still uses positive affirma-

> **When you wake up every morning, tell yourself how well prepared you are to take the NCLEX. Throughout the day, thank yourself for all the hard work you have done. Repeatedly congratulate yourself for how well you are going to score on the test.**

tions to accomplish great things. I want you to also accomplish great things. Give yourself the gift of this tool. Practice it every day, and not just for the NCLEX but for all aspects of your life.

Continue these conversations with yourself throughout the day. Whenever you can, repeat one or two positive affirmation phrases. Write them on post-it paper and put them around the house. They go well on bathroom mirrors, refrigerators, walls, and television screens—and even garage doors! Record a CD of positive affirmations for your car and listen to your voice whenever you are driving.

Practicing these behaviors every day will make an impression in your subconscious mind. You *will* become an empowered test-taker destined for success. Can you feel it yet?

I have encouraged all the students I have tutored over the years not only to do this as a way to help boost themselves psychologically and emotionally and to help them overcome fear, but to also decrease their levels of stress and anxiety. Item writers for the NCLEX are not interested in testing your stress or anxiety. They want to test your knowledge of nursing curriculum, and your ability to critically think, prioritize and problem solve. You are wise to do whatever you can to decrease your stress and anxiety beforehand.

Make a positive affirmation the last thought you have before going to bed at night and the first thought you have when you wake in the morning.

I am prepared for this test.
I have worked hard for this test.
I have scored high on the test.
I will soon be a licensed nurse.
I deserve the high score I will receive on the test.
I will do great things as a nurse.
I am worthwhile and competent.
I am intelligent and ready for this test.
I am confident.
I am proud of myself.
I can remember what I have learned.
I will accomplish great things.
I am a strong client advocate.

STRATEGY

Eliminating fear of the unknown and practicing positive affirmations will aid in reducing stress and anxiety.

ADDITIONAL TEST-TAKING TACTICS

In addition to the test-taking skills and strategies found in Chapter 3 and the 5-Step Approach found in Chapter 4, here is a compilation of additional tactics that many students have found helpful. Try them all. You have nothing to lose.

STRATEGY

Remember that the hospital/clinic settings referred to in the NCLEX questions present ideal situations. You are expected to suppose that staffing is adequate, necessary equipment is available, and resources are attainable. Unless the question directs you to suppose otherwise, picture the ideal situation for the nurse to intervene.

STRATEGY

Remember that the NCLEX is designed to test *your* knowledge, skill, and proficiency, so use caution when choosing an answer that directs the nurse to call the physician, nursing supervisor, or social worker. Make sure you determine that the situation presented in the question cannot be resolved by the nurse. This is accomplished by having an adequate understanding of the scope of practice for the RN or LPN

STRATEGY

Be careful not to make the nurses in your answer superheroes. Know when to delegate and when to act. Again, knowing your scope of practice is imperative.

STRATEGY

When presented with multiple clients in a clinical scenario, immediately determine which client would be your priority. Remember, use the ABCs from Chapter 1 as your guide in determining what client requires attention first. This is the client that will have a nurse assigned to him or her.

STRATEGY

Evaluate the most stable client presented in the scenario. This is the client that most likely can be assessed last or assigned to the nursing assistant or UAP.

STRATEGY

Remember that nurses assess, diagnose, establish goals, intervene, evaluate, and make decisions based on what is needed for our clients. Nurses are educated to complete these tasks. Do not choose answers that have unlicensed personnel performing nursing functions.

STRATEGY

Remember that nurses are the primary teachers and documenters in the hospital and clinic setting. It is rarely advisable to delegate teaching or documentation to others.

STRATEGY

Never choose an answer that reflects dishonesty, inaccuracy, or irrelevance. Sometimes options like these are included in the answers to persuade the test-taker to consider using trickery or coercion as a means of helping a client. Answers such as these are known as distracters. Their purpose is to pull your attention away from the correct information, and are never the right answer.

STRATEGY

Do not change your answer once you have reached a decision. Respect the process you have gone through to come to a conclusion and then stick with it. Although an answer cannot be changed once a question leaves the computer screen, test-takers sometimes lament the option they choose and delay finishing the test. If you use the 5-Step Approach and incorporate skills and strategies into formulating your answer, try not to doubt yourself. I often tell my students when taking a paper and pencil test to remove the eraser from the pencil. The temptation to change answers is then reduced. Remember, do everything you can to be **positive and self-assured.**

STRATEGY

Remember, the NCLEX is a large national test databank, and therefore you will not see patterns to the answers. You cannot surmise that because you have not chosen a "4" for the correct answer in a while that you should do so on the next few questions. The selection of the questions is random and, hence, the answers are also.

STRATEGY

Remember to make a checklist of what you need to bring with you on the day of the test. Include the required identification, snacks, papers, and directions. Do not take any study materials with you: you know, the materials you put away the night before! Instead, take your positive affirmations and re-read them.

NUTRITIONAL PREPARATION

Now that you can see the testing area in your mind and are repeating positive affirmations to yourself, next you need to address your nutritional needs. You should help to make not only your mind better able to function, but also your physical body. This next section is hard for many of my students, but I cannot overemphasize its importance. On the day *before* the test I want you to consume very specific foods, in the morning for breakfast, in the afternoon for lunch, and in the evening for dinner. I want you to eat foods that are rich in protein and moderately high in carbohydrates. Of course, it goes without saying that the menu suggested here is only for those test-takers who have no dietary restrictions.

STRATEGY

I want you to *avoid the use of all alcohol, sugars, stimulants, and caffeine the day and night before, and the morning of, the test*. Eating properly before the test gives you energy that is lasting.

You want to avoid spiking your blood sugar by eating sugary products and sweets. You also want to avoid ingesting any substance that will create elevated physical sensations that decrease over time.

STRATEGY

Another hard request is that you *stop studying* at 6 p.m. the night before your test. At 6 p.m. I want you to close your books and tell yourself that you are ready. Assure yourself that you have done everything you needed to do to prepare for this test.

I ask you to go to bed between 10 p.m. and 11 p.m. and get a good night's sleep. In the morning, you will feel refreshed and ready for the day. Remember to start with positive affirmations and a wholesome breakfast. And do not open a study book. As an educator, it is very upsetting to see my students looking at their notes, reading their books, and cramming, as they call it, just before an exam. Psychologically, when you do this or when you study all night just before the test, you give yourself an unconscious message that you are *not* ready. This kind of behavior can do a lot of damage.

STRATEGY

You should fill your subconscious mind with healthy thoughts of preparedness and tell your subconscious that you are ready to take this test because you have worked hard.

By closing your book at 6 p.m. the night before, going to sleep between 10 p.m. and 11 p.m, and getting a good nights rest, you demonstrate confidence in yourself.

When you wake up in the morning, do not open up a book but rather tell yourself that you are prepared. Confirm your positive affirmations by saying out loud that you will be successful. Then enjoy a breakfast high in protein and moderately high in carbohydrates. Afterward, pack a lunch for yourself consisting of the same types of foods. This will help you to attain and maintain an acceptable level of energy throughout the testing day. I remember when my children were in elementary school, not once did I receive a call from a teacher saying they were tired or sleepy. This was because I never gave them sugary cereals or sweets for breakfast. Instead, they ate eggs, toast and cheese, bagels, leftover chicken, or cold pasta. They had energy that lasted all day long without the influence of sugar and stimulants. Try it. You have nothing to lose, except a mid-day slump.

BE A LONER FOR A DAY

Sometimes being alone can be a good thing.

STRATEGY

I want you to be a loner for a day when you go to test.

I want you to speak with no one. After going to sleep the night before I want you to speak with no one except the family you live with. Speak with no one but the receptionist or proctor at the test site. Speak with no one during the test. Speak with no one if you take a break or if you go to the bathroom or if you stop to have something to eat. The reason I say this is because if you talk to someone about the test or a particular question or a specific topic, you could be convinced that you are not ready to pass the test or that you are not doing well. If you speak with someone at the center who is taking the test with you and they happen to describe a question similar to one you answered, they may share with you that they chose an answer different from your choice. Expectedly, your first thought might be that you got the question **wrong**. That one thought can chip away at your self-confidence; that one thought can reach into your subconscious mind and say you are not doing well. An innocent comment can cause you to believe that you should have studied more. Thoughts such as these are confidence killers and will only do you harm.

Have lunch alone. Take a break by yourself. Keep your thoughts positive and do not let anyone's words harm your self-esteem or bring your high spirits down. If you stay alone, no one can make you believe you are not ready. Repeat your positive affirmations in your mind over and over again.

STRATEGY **Do yourself another huge favor and *turn your cell phone or pager off at 10 p.m. the night before and do not turn it on again until after the test.***

I understand this is a big request but it is an important one. After you have completed the test, call whomever you want. I also want to discourage you from carpooling to the test. Carpooling encourages conversations, and talking about the test is inevitable. This topic of conversation can hurt your subconscious mind and again make you believe you are not ready.

It is vital that you practice positive affirmations every day. During the test, tell yourself you can hear your nursing professor lecture; you can read your textbook; and you can see the notes you took in class. Psychologically and emotionally, do everything you can to fill yourself with positive thoughts. See yourself as a licensed practical nurse or as a licensed registered professional nurse. See yourself practicing nursing in a hospital or other health care setting. See yourself working side by side with physicians and other nurses. Recall these mental images whenever needed during the test to keep your confidence up.

STRATEGY

When you walk into the test center *check your stress, your nerves, and your anxiety at the door.*

Practice deep breathing exercises and relaxation techniques. These can be very beneficial when taking a test. Concentrate on your breathing and every time you breathe in, tell yourself you are filling with confidence. Every time you exhale, understand you are blowing away doubt and anxiety. Now, breathe in deeply and inhale confidence for all that hard work you have done. Now, exhale and blow away the doubt, the tension, the fear, and the anxiety.

> **Breathe in confidence and exhale doubt and anxiety.**

I also recommend that you practice relaxation techniques. Often before an exam I ask my students to sit in a comfortable position with their eyes closed. Practice along with me. Sit comfortably and close your eyes. As you do this, start concentrating on relaxing the muscles of your head, the muscles of your face, and then the muscles in your neck. Move down your shoulders, down your arms, over your stomach, and down your back. Continue relaxing down your legs, ankles, feet, and toes. Just relax and feel all the tension leave. Once you are in a relaxed state, remind yourself how well you know the 5-Step Approach and how it will work for you. Reinforce to yourself that you know the skills and strategies, and will use them to help you pass the test.

Practice makes things, such as building confidence, become part of us, and you can bring this confidence with you when you go to test. If you read the testimonials in Chapter 1 and at the end of this chapter, you can begin to understand how important physical and emotional preparation can be. Once you have completed the intellectual preparation presented in this book and you have worked hard to answer all the questions using the 5-Step Approach and to master the skills and strategies that I have collected over the years, you are nearing the end of your NCLEX preparation. An additional request I have is for you to think of including exercise and fresh air into your daily routine. Start by making it a habit of going outside to get some fresh air every day. Take a walk or climb an extra set of stairs. Do some reading and practice relaxing. Allay your fears and decrease your tension and anxiety. Most importantly, continue to fill yourself with confidence. Congratulations on a job well done!

Student Profile 3

"I met Dr. DiDona 3 years ago through a mutual friend. I was shy and quiet but I began tutoring with her and found her skills and strategies very helpful. I made a commitment to use the 5-Step Approach and I was ready to test in a matter of weeks. I prepared myself just like she told me. I drove to the test site a few days before the test. I went inside and looked around. I think the proctor thought I was a little strange but I didn't care. I went into the bathroom and walked around the parking lot. I ate the foods Dr. DiDona recommended the day before and the day of the test. And I spoke to NO ONE! That was really hard for me but I was able to keep my level of confidence very high. I passed. I was so proud of myself. I hadn't told anyone I was testing so my family was surprised.

"All I can say is try using the 5-Step Approach and the skills and strategies. You have nothing to lose and everything to gain. I feel I can say with certainty that this book will be the most important tool you can use as you prepare for the NCLEX. Use it over and over again, reference it, and study it. I found Dr. DiDona's techniques unlike any other teacher I had in nursing school. Thanks, Dr. D."

Anonymous Nurse

1. A client is returned to your surgical unit from the postanesthesia care unit in skeletal traction. The nurse assesses the client and takes action to correct which of the following problems with the traction setup?

    1. The ropes are knotted and centered in the wheel grooves.
    2. The weights are resting against the foot of the bed.
    3. The weights are evenly matched on each side.
    4. The ropes are securely attached to the pin.

    Answer: 2

    Rationale: Weights that are resting against the foot of the bed or on the floor do not allow the traction apparatus to do its job. The ropes should be knotted and attached to the pin and in the center of the wheel grooves. The weights should be evenly matched on each side.

    Client Need: Physiological Integrity

2. A client has been diagnosed with a gastric ulcer and has been ordered Carafate 1 g by mouth four times a day. The nurse understands that teaching was effective in the use of this medication when the client states which of the following?

    1. "I will take my medicine every 4 hours around the clock."
    2. "I will take my medicine after meals and at bedtime."
    3. "I will take my medicine with meals and when I wake up in the morning."
    4. "I will take my medicine 1 hour before meals and at bedtime."

    Answer: 4

    Rationale: Carafate should be administered 1 hour before meals and at bedtime. This allows the medication to coat the ulcer to prevent irritation by food intake. Answers 1, 2, and 3 are incorrect.

    Did you use Bs and Gs to find the correct answer?

    Client Need: Physiological Integrity

3.   A client comes to the emergency room via ambulance with complaints of severe radiating chest pain and shortness of breath. The client is restless, frightened, and slightly cyanotic. The house physician's orders include oxygen by nasal cannula at 4 l/min stat, cardiac enzyme levels, intravenous fluids, and a 12-lead electrocardiogram. Which of the following nursing actions is a priority for the nurse to take **first**?

1.   Attach client to a 12-lead electrocardiogram.
2.   Draw the blood and send it to the lab.
3.   Apply the oxygen into the client.
4.   Start the intravenous line.

Answer: 3

Rationale: The priority nursing intervention is to apply oxygen because the client is most likely experiencing myocardial ischemia. The client will have an electrocardiogram, blood drawn, and an intravenous line started, but these are not the priority interventions.

> Did you remember the ABCs? Airway is the priority.

Client Need: Physiological Integrity

4.   A labor and delivery room nurse admits a woman who is 38 weeks gestation and in early labor. Admission assessment is completed, and the nurse discovers the mother's temperature is 102°F. What is the nurse's **most** appropriate nursing action?

1.   Document the finding and recheck the client's temperature in 4 hours.
2.   Administer Tylenol as ordered and recheck the temperature in 30 minutes.
3.   Notify the client's physician.
4.   Place the client on a hyperthermia blanket.

Answer: 3

Rationale: A client in early labor with a fever of 102°F may be experiencing an infection. The priority is to address the infection as quickly as possible. The physician needs to be notified so that orders may be given to the nurse. Documenting the finding, administering Tylenol to reduce the fever, and placing the client on a hyperthermia blanket are not the priorities in this situation.

Client Need: Physiological Integrity

5.   A client with active tuberculosis is admitted to your unit. The nurse assigns the client to a bed based on the knowledge that which of the following protocol must be followed?

1. All clients with active tuberculosis are admitted to four-bed rooms.
2. The client with active tuberculosis is admitted to a two-bed room with another nonsurgical client.
3. Clients with active tuberculosis are admitted to private rooms that are well ventilated and have a minimum of six air exchanges per hour.
4. The client will be immediately transferred to the intensive care unit.

Answer: 3

Rationale: Clients with active tuberculosis are not put into rooms with other clients. They are placed on respiratory isolation in private rooms that are well ventilated with a minimum of six air exchanges each hour that are ventilated to the outside.

> Did you notice the word "all" in answer 1? Eliminate this option.

Client Need: Safe Effective Care Environment

6.   A 6-month-old infant is admitted with a diagnosis of suspected hydrocephalus. Which of the following signs and symptoms would the nurse expect to assess in an infant with this diagnosis?

1. Proteinuria.
2. Hypotension.
3. Tachycardia.
4. Bulging anterior fontanel.

Answer: 4

Rationale: A bulging anterior fontanel is a sign and symptom of increased amounts of cerebral spinal fluid and is a classic sign and symptom of hydrocephalus. Proteinuria, hypotension, and tachycardia are not associated with hydrocephalus.

Client Need: Physiological Integrity

7. A client comes to the healthcare clinic complaining of low back pain. He states that his wife has encouraged him to exercise. He asks the nurse which exercises would be best for him to participate in. The nurse knows that which of the following exercises are most beneficial for this client's low back pain?

1. Tennis.
2. Canoeing.
3. Swimming.
4. Archery.

Answer: 3

Rationale: Exercises such as swimming and walking can be very beneficial for clients with low back pain. These types of exercises help to strengthen back muscles. Tennis, canoeing, and archery may cause strain and therefore increase lower back pain.

Client Need: Health Promotion and Maintenance

8. A 4-year-old child is being discharged from the hospital after having a myringotomy with tubes inserted. The mother asks the nurse what to do if the tubes fall out. The nurse correctly instructs the mother to do which of the following?

1. Replace the tubes immediately into the ears.
2. Take the child without delay to the emergency room.
3. Call the health care clinic and report that the tubes have fallen out.
4. Reassure the mother that the tubes will not fall out.

Answer: 3

Rationale: It is important that the mother be reassured that the tubes falling out is not considered an emergency but that the child's surgeon needs to be notified. The mother should be instructed not to attempt to reinsert the tubes. It is wrong for the nurse to reassure the mother that the tubes will not fall out. There is no need for the child to be taken to the emergency room.

Client Need: Physiological Integrity

9. A 47-year-old woman has been diagnosed with cervical cancer. The physician has instructed the client to come in for laser surgery in an outpatient setting. The nurse completes the preoperative teaching. Which statement, if made by the client to the nurse, indicates that the client understands the purpose of laser surgery?

1. "My cancer is too extensive for traditional surgery."
2. "Laser surgery is the only way to remove my cancer."
3. "My surgeon can see the edges of my cancer clearly."
4. "Laser surgery ensures my cancer will not come back."

Answer: 3

Rationale: Laser surgery is a very useful method for removing cervical cancer when the surgeon can clearly visualize all edges of the lesion. Answers 1, 2, and 4 are inappropriate.

Did you use 3 Bs and 1 G?

Client Need: Physiological Integrity

10. The physician orders a particular medication to be administered intravenously every 6 hours. The dosage of the medication is 650 mg. The medication label reads 2 g to be reconstituted with 5 ml of sterile water. What is the amount of medication the nurse will draw in preparation to administer one dose?

1. 0.62 ml.
2. 2.0 ml.
3. 1.62 ml.
4. 2.2 ml.

Answer: 3

Rationale: The first thing to do is to convert 2 g to 2000 mg. The formula to use is the doctor's order divided by the available dose multiplied by the volume. This would leave 650 mg divided by 2000 mg multiplied by 5 ml. The answer is 1.62 ml.

Client Need: Physiological Integrity

11. A nursing instructor is reviewing with a group of nursing students how to care for a child with sickle cell disease who is suffering from an acute occlusive crisis. Which statement, if made by the nursing student, indicates to the nursing instructor a need for further instruction?

1. "I know my client will need intravenous fluids for hydration."
2. "I will administer a Motrin tablet to my client if needed to manage the pain."
3. "I will offer the child fluids by mouth frequently."
4. "I will administer oxygen to the child as ordered by the physician."

Answer: 2

Rationale: A child with sickle cell disease experiencing an acute occlusive crisis would be managed with strong narcotic analgesics, such as morphine sulfate. Motrin is contraindicated in controlling pain associated with a sickle cell crisis. Intravenous fluids and oral hydration would be a part of the child's care plan. Oxygen administration is an appropriate nursing intervention.

Client Need: Physiological Integrity

Did you try using step 4 for this question?

---

12. The mother of an adolescent male client calls the psychiatric health clinic and tells the nurse she believes her teenage son is at risk for suicide. Which statement, if made by the mother, indicates to the nurse that the adolescent may be contemplating suicide?

1. The mother tells the nurse that her son plans to use his belt to hang himself in the shower.
2. The adolescent refuses to visit with his friends.
3. The adolescent spends most of his time locked in his room.
4. The mother tells the nurse she hears her son crying for hours on end.

Answer: 1

Rationale: A client who has a plan for suicide and is able to share that plan must be taken seriously. The mother should be instructed to initiate suicide precautions. Answers 2, 3, and 4 demonstrate that the adolescent is depressed but do not indicate a plan or intention for suicide.

Did answer 1 stand alone? Step 4 is applicable for this question.

Client Need: Psychosocial Integrity

---

13. A client is admitted to your unit with a diagnosis of diabetes mellitus. The physician orders the client to have 25 units of NPH insulin every morning if the client's blood glucose level is greater than 200 mg/dl. The nurse knows to monitor this client for signs and symptoms of hypoglycemia because NPH insulin peaks in how many hours after administration?

1. 1 hour.
2. 3 to 4 hours.
3. 5 to 12 hours.
4. 8 to 16 hours.

Answer: 3

Rationale: NPH insulin is an intermediate-acting insulin. The onset of NPH is 3 to 4 hours. The duration of NPH is 18 to 28 hours. The peak time for NPH is 5 to 12 hours.

> **Step 5 works well with this question.**

Client Need: Physiological Integrity

---

14.   A nursing instructor is lecturing a group of nursing students about families experiencing violence. Which of the following statements, if made by a nursing student, indicates to the nursing instructor a need for further teaching?

1. "Men who abuse women usually have poor self-esteem."
2. "Abusers like to use fear and intimidation on their victims."
3. "Men who are abusers are usually immature and dependent on others."
4. "Abusers usually come from low-income families."

Answer: 4

Rationale: Men and women who are abusers come from all socioeconomic levels. Abusers typically do have poor self-esteem, immaturity, and demonstrate dependence. Fear and intimidation are tactics often used by abusers.

> **Did you try using "bad" and "good" for this teaching question?**

Client Need: Psychosocial Integrity

---

15.   A client comes to the outpatient clinic to have an intravenous cholangiogram. He has been diagnosed with cholelithiasis and has been in pain for 1 week. The nurse prepares the client for the procedure by teaching him the purpose of the test. Which statement, if made by the client, indicates to the nurse that teaching was understood?

1. "They are going to examine my gallbladder and ducts."
2. "They are going to remove my gallstones."
3. "They are going to wash out my gallbladder."
4. "They are going to put medication into my gallbladder."

Answer: 1

Rationale: An intravenous cholangiogram is a test used for diagnostic purposes only. It enables the physician to look at the gallbladder and the surrounding ducts. It is not used to remove gallstones, wash out the gallbladder, or instill medication.

> Did answer 1 stand alone as the only assessment procedure? Answers 2, 3, and 4 include interventions.

Client Need: Physiological Integrity

16. A woman who is 38 weeks gestation comes to the hospital in active labor. The client is positive for human immunodeficiency virus (HIV). The nurse knows that an important goal for this client is to prevent the transmission of HIV to the fetus. To aid in the prevention of transmission of HIV, the nurse would expect the obstetrician to order all of the following **except**

1. Epidural anesthesia.
2. An internal intrauterine pressure catheter.
3. Pitocin intravenously.
4. Direct internal fetal heart rate monitoring.

Answer: 4

Rationale: It is important for obstetricians to use caution during the intrapartum period for clients who are HIV positive. To help decrease the risk of transmission of HIV to the fetus, the obstetrician would not order direct fetal heart rate monitoring unless necessary. Epidural anesthesia,

Pitocin intravenously, and an internal intrauterine pressure catheter would not place the fetus at risk.

Client Need: Safe Effective Care Environment

> **Did you associate the need for fetal safety in the question to the fetal intervention in the answer?**

---

17.   A nursing student is learning to auscultate breath sounds on clients. The nursing instructor asked the nursing student which part of the stethoscope is to be placed directly on the client's skin. The nursing student correctly answers _____.

Answer: The diaphragm

Rationale: To correctly auscultate breath sounds the nursing student should apply the diaphragm of the stethoscope directly to the client's skin. The bell of the stethoscope is not used for this.

Client Need: Health Promotion and Maintenance

---

18.   A visiting nurse is in the home of a 78-year-old woman. The client tells the nurse that she is feeling tired and is unable to grocery shop. The client asks the nurse if she could pick up a few things at a local store. Which of the following responses would be *best* for the nurse to make?

1. "It is against policy for me to grocery shop for you."
2. "I would be happy to do whatever I could to help you."
3. "Nurses don't have time to grocery shop and besides I have a bad back."
4. "It's unfortunate you don't have someone to help you on the days you don't feel well. Let's talk about how we can solve that for you."

Answer: 4

Rationale: It is inappropriate for a nurse to refuse to help a client without offering assistance with the cause of the problem. It is also inappropriate for a nurse to volunteer to go grocery shopping while ignoring the cause of the problem. Nurses should not share personal health information. Acknowledging that the client needs assistance on certain days and offering to find a solution for that problem are most beneficial for the client.

Did you notice that number 4 was the most comprehensive answer?

Client Need: Psychosocial Integrity

---

19. A client is admitted to the hospital and placed on seizure precautions. The nurse knows that it is important for client safety to include all the following nursing interventions **except** to

1. Stay in the client's room while the client is showering.
2. Keep the client's bed in the lowest position.
3. Keep all lights on in the client's room while sleeping.
4. Assist the client to ambulate in the hallway.

Answer: 3

Rationale: It is important for the nurse to monitor the client while the client is showering, to keep the client's bed in the lowest position, and to assist the client in ambulating. It is not appropriate to keep all lights on in the room while the client is sleeping. Part of seizure precautions is to provide the client with a quiet and restful environment.

Did you notice the word "all" in answer 3? That should have told you the statement was incorrect, and the question was asking for an incorrect statement.

Client Need: Safe Effective Care Environment

---

20. A 60-year-old man involved in a motor vehicle accident is in the intensive care unit and needs mechanical ventilation for support. After 3 days the nurse determines that the client's condition has improved. Which of the following, if observed by the nurse, indicates there is respiratory improvement?

1. The client has a decreased need for supplemental oxygen.
2. The client is experiencing tachypnea.
3. The client's breath sounds are unequal bilaterally.
4. The client's arterial blood gas levels show an increase in CO_2 in the blood.

Answer: 1

Rationale: The client's decreased need for supplemental oxygen is a positive sign of improvement. Tachypnea, unequal breath sounds bilaterally, and an increase in the serum CO_2 level are indications of the client's condition worsening.

Client Need: Physiological Integrity

21. The nurse is caring for a client in the cardiac care unit. The client has arterial blood gases drawn. The client's pH is 7.3 and the $PaCO_2$ is 50. The nurse correctly determines that the client has _____.

Answer: Respiratory acidosis

Rationale: In clients with respiratory acidosis, the pH level is decreased and the $PaCO_2$ level is elevated.

Client Need: Physiological Integrity

22. A newly delivered client has a positive Homans' sign, and the nurse correctly suspects deep vein thrombosis. Which nursing action is the **priority** for the nurse to include in the client's plan of care?

1. Elevation of the affected extremity.
2. Ice packs applied to the affected calf.
3. Active range of motion exercises every 2 hours.
4. Calf measurements every 4 hours.

Answer: 1

Rationale: Standard interventions for a client diagnosed with deep vein thrombosis include bed rest, elevation of the affected extremity, and the application of warm moist soaks. Active range of motion is discouraged because of the risk of dislodging the clot and causing a pulmonary embolism. Calf measurements may be included and should be done on a daily basis.

Client Need: Physiological Integrity

---

23.   An elderly client diagnosed with rheumatoid arthritis has aspirin grains 10 orally every 4 hours PRN ordered. On hand are 325-mg aspirin tablets. How many tablets should the nurse administer?

_____

Answer: 2

Rationale: The formula used in this equation is desired dose divided by dose on hand and multiplied by the quantity. Hence, 10 grains is converted to 600 mg. 600 mg is divided by 325 mg and multiplied by one tablet. The answer is 2 tablets.

> Did you remember not to label your answer? The label was included in the question.

Client Need: Physiological Integrity

---

24.   The pediatric nurse is caring for a child with a tracheostomy. The nurse suction's the child's tracheostomy and determines the effectiveness of the suctioning based on which of the following assessments?

1. The child's respiratory rate is increased.
2. The child's oxygen saturation level is decreased.
3. The child's breath sounds are clear.
4. The child's capillary refill is normal.

Answer: 3

Rationale: The most accurate way of determining if respiratory secretions have been cleared after suctioning is to auscultate breath sounds. The child's respiratory rate should decrease, and the oxygen saturation level should increase. Capillary refill is not associated with breath sounds.

Client Need: Physiological Integrity

25.   A client is scheduled for a bronchoscopy in the late morning. The nurse preparing the client for the procedure would complete all the following nursing interventions *except*

1. Having the client sign an informed consent.
2. Removing all prosthetic devices.
3. Answering any questions the client has about the procedure.
4. Serving the client tea and toast for breakfast.

Answer: 4

Rationale: The client having a bronchoscopy should be NPO for a minimum of 6 hours before the procedure. The client should sign an informed consent, and all prosthetic devices should be removed. The client has the right to have any questions answered.

Client Need: Physiological Integrity

26.   The emergency room nurse is assessing a client who was injured playing tackle football. It is suspected that the client has fractured ribs. Which nursing assessments would be typical of a client with fractured ribs? Select all that apply.

1. Pain on expiration.
2. Pain on inspiration.
3. Deep rapid respirations.
4. Shallow guarded respirations.
5. No change in the client's respirations.

Answers: 2 and 4

Rationale: Clients with fractured ribs typically complain of pain on inspiration as the lungs inflate and demonstrate shallow guarded respirations.

Client Need: Physiological Integrity

---

27. A nurse is caring for a client with a tracheostomy. The nurse is preparing to perform suctioning of the tracheostomy. Which of the following items would the nurse have at the client's bedside?

1. A tracheostomy care kit, suction kit, and sterile saline.
2. A tracheostomy care kit, hydrogen peroxide, and Betadine solution.
3. Sterile water and sterile combine dressings.
4. A tracheostomy care kit, suction catheter, and clean gloves.

Answer: 1

Rationale: A nurse preparing to suction a tracheostomy should have a tracheostomy care kit at the bedside along with sterile saline or sterile water and a sterile suction kit. Betadine solution, combine dressings, and clean gloves are not used in the care and suctioning of a tracheostomy.

> Ah-ha! Did you remember to deep breathe and stretch?

Client Need: Physiological Integrity

---

28. A client has a chest tube removed and is discharged home. The nurse providing home care instructions determines that the client needs further instruction when the client states which of the following?

1. "I will call my doctor if I have any trouble breathing."
2. "I will avoid lifting any heavy objects for at least 6 weeks."
3. "I will watch for any signs of infection."
4. "I will remove the chest tube site dressing as soon as I get home."

Answer: 4

Rationale: A clients who is discharged home after removal of a chest tube should be taught to report any difficulties breathing, avoid lifting heavy objects, and watch for any signs of infection. The client should also be taught **not** to remove the dressing.

Client Need: Health Promotion and Maintenance

29.   A visiting nurse goes to the home of a mother who had a normal vaginal delivery 5 days ago. On assessment, the nurse determines that the client is experiencing breast engorgement. The nurse teaches the mother how to care for this condition. Which of the following statements, if made by the mother, indicates to the nurse that teaching was successful?

1. "I will let my baby breastfeed on only one breast each time."
2. "I will avoid wearing a bra during the daytime."
3. "I will apply cold compresses to my breasts before each feeding."
4. "I will massage my breasts before I feed my baby to stimulate the let-down reflex."

Answer: 4

Rationale: Measures to treat breast engorgement include massaging the breasts before each feeding to stimulate the letdown reflex. Women with breast engorgement should be encouraged to wear a bra at all times and to alternate breasts when feeding. Applying a warm compress and taking a warm shower before breastfeeding also helps to stimulate the letdown reflex.

> Did you notice the words "only" and "cold" in answers 1 and 3? These options should be eliminated.

Client Need: Health Promotion and Maintenance

30.   A client with valvular heart disease is at risk for developing left-sided congestive heart failure. The nurse knows to monitor for which of the following as the most likely indication that the client has developed left-sided congestive heart failure?

1. The apical pulse rate.
2. The client's activity tolerance.
3. The client's breath sounds.
4. The client's blood pressure.

> Did you remember that *l*eft-sided congestive heart failure is characterized by edema of the *l*ungs?

Answer: 3

Rationale: One of the best ways of determining the onset of left-sided congestive heart failure is to auscultate crackles or rails in the lungs. Assessing the client's pulse rate, activity tolerance, and blood pressure are important but are not necessarily indicative of congestive heart failure.

Client Need: Physiological Integrity

31.   A client is admitted with a diagnosis of peptic ulcer disease. The nurse knows to assess the client for signs indicating gastrointestinal perforation. Which of the following is a classic indication of gastrointestinal perforation?

1. Hyperactive bowel sounds.
2. Sudden severe abdominal pain.
3. Positive stool for guaiac.
4. Bounding pulse.

Answer: 2

Rationale: Sudden severe abdominal pain is indicative of gastrointestinal perforation. When perforation occurs, the client will also experience a rigid abdomen. The bowel sounds will decrease, and the pulse will weaken. Stools that test positive for blood are not indicative of a perforation.

Client Need: Physiological Integrity

32. A client diagnosed with chronic anxiety is being discharged from the psychiatric unit. The nurse develops a plan of care for the client that includes which of the following appropriate goals? The client will

1. Contact the crisis counselor once a week.
2. Identify anxiety-producing situations.
3. Ignore feelings of anxiety and think happy thoughts.
4. Eliminate all stress and anxiety from daily life.

Answer: 2

Rationale: A crisis counselor should be contacted when needed. Ignoring feelings of anxiety and asking the client to think happy thoughts is unrealistic. It is not possible to eliminate **all** stress and anxiety from daily life.

Client Need: Psychosocial Integrity

> Did you notice the word "all" in option 4 and eliminate that answer?

33. An emergency room nurse is caring for a client brought in with severe chest pain. Within minutes the client becomes pulseless and loses consciousness. What piece of equipment would the nurse obtain immediately for the care of this client?

1. A blood pressure cuff.
2. An electrocardiogram machine.
3. An external pacemaker.
4. A cardiac defibrillator.

Answer: 4

Rationale: A client who becomes pulseless and loses consciousness must be defibrillated quickly. In the absence of a defibrillator, the nurse would begin performing cardiopulmonary resuscitation. A blood pressure cuff, electrocardiogram machine, and external pacemaker may all be used but are not the priority piece of equipment.

Client Need: Physiological Integrity

34.   A client on a psychiatric ward suddenly becomes violent and is placed in a seclusion room. As the client is secluded, the nurse should do which of the following?

1. Not speak to the client.
2. Tell the client to be calm and seclusion will be short.
3. Ask the client why he became violent.
4. Inform the client that he is being secluded to help regain self-control.

Answer: 4

Rationale: A client who suddenly becomes violent and needs to be secluded should be informed of the purpose of seclusion. Not speaking to the client, telling the client to be calm, and asking the client why he became violent are punitive actions.

Client Need: Psychosocial Integrity

35.   A nursery nurse administers the first dose of hepatitis B vaccine to a newborn infant. The mother asks the nurse if her baby needs further hepatitis B immunizations. Which response by the nurse is most informative for the mother regarding hepatitis B immunization scheduling?

1. "Your baby should have a second immunization between the ages of 1 and 2 months and a final immunization 4 months after the initial dose."
2. "Your baby needs a second hepatitis B immunization when he is 6 months of age and a third immunization at 1 year of age."
3. "Your baby can receive one more hepatitis B immunization anytime after his first birthday."
4. "Your baby only needs this one hepatitis B vaccine injection."

Answer: 1

Rationale: The most recent vaccination schedule for infants who receive hepatitis B vaccines are zero months or at the time of birth, at 1 to 2 months of age, and then at 4 months after the initial dose. Answers 2, 3, and 4 are incorrect.

Client Need: Health Promotion and Maintenance

36.   A child is admitted to the hospital with a diagnosis of rheumatic fever. The nurse is questioning the mother and includes which information in the initial assessment?

1. The child has not experienced dysuria.
2. The child's sister had a sore throat 2 weeks ago.
3. The child's father had an intestinal flu last month.
4. The next-door neighbor's child has chickenpox.

Answer: 2

Rationale: Rheumatic fever typically presents 2 to 6 weeks after the child has experienced an untreated or improperly treated streptococcal infection of the respiratory tract. Answers 1, 3, and 4 are unrelated to the assessment findings of rheumatic fever.

Client Need: Physiological Integrity

37.   A nursing instructor is teaching a nursing student about caring for clients diagnosed with anemia. The nursing instructor knows that a good source of dietary iron that the body can readily absorb is which of the following food items?

1. Green leafy vegetables.
2. Fresh fruits.
3. Chicken.
4. Whole grain cereals.

Answer: 3

Rationale: Many foods are considered dietary sources of iron, including meat,

> **Did you remember to choose chicken as a nutritionally superior food item?**

vegetables, fruits, and cereals. Chicken is the easiest source of iron for the body to absorb.

Client Need: Health Promotion and Maintenance

---

38.   A school nurse is teaching a class of students about sexually transmitted diseases (STDs). The nurse knows that teaching was effective when a student makes the following statement:

1. "I will take birth control pills to protect myself from STDs."
2. "I will use a diaphragm to prevent an STD."
3. "I will tell my boyfriend that using a condom is all the protection we need."
4. "I know that not having sex with multiple partners can help prevent STDs."

Answer: 4

Rationale: Birth control pills and diaphragms do not help in the prevention of STDs. Condoms do provide some protection, but not having casual sex with multiple partners is a primary way of preventing STDs.

> Did you notice the word "all" in answer 3? It should be eliminated immediately.

Client Need: Safe Effective Care Environment

---

39.   The nurse is caring for a newly delivered mother on a postpartum unit after a cesarean birth. The nurse documents which intervention in the client's plan of care that will assist in the prevention of thrombophlebitis?

1. Apply warm moist soaks to the client's lower legs.
2. Keep the client on bed rest with the lower legs elevated.
3. Apply support stockings to the client before getting out of bed.
4. Have the client ambulate frequently in the hallway.

Answer: 4

Rationale: Venous stasis is believed to be a major cause of the development of thrombophlebitis. It is advisable for the newly delivered cesarean section client to ambulate as early as possible and as frequently as she can. There is no indication for the client to have warm moist soaks or to apply support hose. Bed rest is contraindicated for this client.

Client Need: Physiological Integrity

40. A 35-year-old woman has a history of fibrocystic disease of the breasts. The nurse caring for this client determines that the client understands the nature of the disorder when the client states that her signs and symptoms will most likely occur at what time of the month?

　　1. Before her menses begins.
　　2. After her menses ends.
　　3. In the winter months.
　　4. In the hot summer months.

Answer: 1

Rationale: The client with fibrocystic breast disease understands the disorder when she states that symptoms are more likely to occur before the onset of menses. These symptoms include painful breasts, smooth moveable lumps, and possible nipple discharge. Answers 2, 3, and 4 are incorrect.

Client Need: Physiological Integrity

41. A 50-year-old man returns to unit from the postanesthesia care unit (PACU) after a transurethral resection of the prostate (TURP). The client has a three-way Foley catheter inserted in his bladder. The nurse assessing the client would be alert for urine that is which color?

1. Pink.
2. Dark pink.
3. Bright red.
4. Amber.

> Did you remember Airway, Breathing, and Circulation to help answer this question? Also, step 5.

Answer: 3

Rationale: Bright red urine indicates bleeding and should be reported to the surgeon immediately. Urine that is pink or amber is not considered to be alarming.

Client Need: Physiological Integrity

---

42. A 52-year-old woman returns from the operating room after a left mastectomy with axillary lymph node dissection. After an uneventful stay in the hospital, the nurse completes discharge teaching. The nurse determines that the client understands postoperative instructions and arm care if the client states which of the following?

1. "I will only use a straight edge razor to shave under my arms."
2. "I will only allow blood pressure to be taken on my left arm."
3. "I will carry my pocketbook and grocery bags using only my left arm."
4. "I will wear gloves whenever I am working in my kitchen."

Answer: 4

Rationale: Clients who have a mastectomy with axillary lymph node dissection are at increased risk for edema and infection. The client should be taught to avoid activities that increase edema or may cause damage, such as carrying heavy objects and having blood pressures taken on the affected arm. Wearing gloves and using pot holders are recommended to prevent injury.

> Did you notice the word "only" in answers 1, 2, and 3?

Client Need: Health Promotion and Maintenance

43. A nurse is teaching a class of senior citizens in the community center on the prevention of colorectal cancer. The nurse places the highest priority on reducing the risk factors for developing colorectal cancer, which include which of the following factors?

1. A positive gastrointestinal history.
2. Familial history of colorectal cancer.
3. Age.
4. A diet high in fat and low in fiber.

Answer: 4

Rationale: Risk factors for colorectal cancer that cannot be changed include a past history of gastrointestinal disorders, familial tendencies, and age. Clients should be aware that modifying the diet to low fat and high fiber is preferable.

> Did you take your time reading this question to *really* understand what it asked?

Client Needs: Health Promotion and Maintenance

44. A client in labor receives Stadol for pain. The nurse knows that when administering this medication the priority is to have which medication readily available?

_____

Answer: Narcan.

Rationale: Stadol is classified as an opioid analgesic. The nurse would make sure that Narcan and resuscitation equipment are readily available in the event the client experiences respiratory depression.

Client Need: Physiological Integrity

45. A client is returned to the unit after an endoscopic procedure. What nursing assessment is a priority for the nurse to complete after checking the client's vital signs?

1. Monitor the client for pain.
2. Monitor the client for signs of gastrointestinal upset.
3. Assess the client for return of the gag reflex.
4. Allow the client to perform a warm gargle.

Answer: 3

Rationale: The nurse places the highest priority on assessing the client for return of the gag reflex. This is an important part of maintaining the client's airway. Monitoring the client for pain and for gastrointestinal upset is not the priority. The client would not be allowed to gargle until the gag reflex has returned.

Client Need: Physiological Integrity

46. A nurse is preparing to administer medication to a client diagnosed with myasthenia gravis. Before administering medications, the nurse would ask the client to perform which priority action?

1. Empty the client's bladder.
2. Put up the side rails on the bed.
3. Take a few sips of water.
4. Place the client in a low Fowler's position.

Answer: 3

Rationale: The priority intervention is to determine the client's ability to swallow. Clients who are diagnosed with myasthenia gravis often have an inability to swallow. Answers 1, 2, and 4 are not associated with clients who have myasthenia gravis.

Client Need: Safe Effective Care Environment

47.   A client is suffering from chronic pain and has decided to use a transcutaneous electrical nerve stimulation device (TENs) as prescribed by his physician for the relief of chronic pain. The nurse has taught the client about the use and purpose of the TENs unit. Which of the following statements, if made by the client, indicates to the nurse there is a need for further teaching?

    1.   "I wish I didn't have to attach the electrodes to my skin."
    2.   "It's unfortunate I have to be in the hospital for this treatment."
    3.   "I am happy. This unit will help relieve my pain."
    4.   "I hope I don't have to take as many pain pills."

Answer: 2

Rationale: The TENs unit is designed to be portable and to be controlled by the client. There is no need for the client to be in the hospital. The client does need to have electrodes attached to his skin. The client should experience less pain and take less pain medication.

Client Need: Physiological Integrity

48.   A client has a cast applied to the lower leg as a result of a bone fracture. The next day the client returns complaining of irritated skin around the edge of the cast. Which nursing intervention is a priority for the nurse to complete?

    1.   Give the client cream to apply to the irritated skin.
    2.   Have the client massage the skin around the cast twice a day.
    3.   Have the client use talcum powder on the irritated skin.
    4.   Petal the edges of the cast with tape.

Answer: 4

Rationale: Petaling the edges of a cast with tape helps to minimize skin irritation. The client should never put anything down the sides of the cast.

> **Did you notice that answer 4 deals with the *cause* of the discomfort?**

Client Need: Physiological Integrity

49. A client on cardiac medications and diuretics comes to the clinic to have a serum potassium level drawn. The results show the client's potassium level is 6.1 mEq/l. This result should prompt the nurse to take which of the following priority actions?

    1. Contact the client's physician.
    2. Draw blood for a serum sodium level.
    3. Encourage the client to increase fluid intake by mouth.
    4. Do nothing, as this level is within normal limits.

Answer: 1

Rationale: A serum potassium level of 6.1 mEq/l is dangerously high and could cause cardiac dysrhythmias and potentially cardiac arrest. Because of this risk, the physician must be notified immediately. Checking the client's sodium level and encouraging extra fluids by mouth will not resolve an elevated potassium level.

Client Need: Physiological Integrity

50. A newborn infant is admitted to the neonatal intensive care unit. On admission, the nurse notices that the newborn's internal viscera are located outside of the abdominal cavity and not covered with a sack. The nurse anticipates the physician to diagnose the newborn with _____.

Answer: Gastroschisis

Rationale: Gastroschisis is a defect of the abdominal wall in newborns where the internal viscera are located outside of the abdomen without a sack. Immediate surgery is required.

Did you remember how to spell gastroschisis? Keep in mind that spelling counts.

Client Need: Physiological Integrity

51. A client is admitted to the intensive care unit with a diagnosis of pulmonary embolism. The nurse implements which of the following physician orders immediately?

   1. Administer morphine sulfate intravenously.
   2. Administer oxygen therapy as ordered.
   3. Start an intravenous line of Ringer's lactate.
   4. Place the client on a cardiac monitor.

Answer: 2

Rationale: The client with a pulmonary embolism requires oxygen therapy immediately because of the risk of hypoxemia. Very often pulmonary edema is associated with respiratory distress and cyanosis. Administering morphine sulfate, starting an intravenous line, and placing the client on a cardiac monitor will all be done, but they are not the priority nursing interventions.

> **Did you remember your ABCs (airway, breathing, and circulation)? Oxygen is the priority need for this client.**

Client Need: Physiological Integrity

52. The nurse is caring for a young woman diagnosed with metastatic carcinoma. The client tells the nurse she is angry and that she does not want to learn how to treat her illness because she knows she cannot be cured. Based on this client's statement, the nurse determines that the client is experiencing which potential problem?

   1. Impairment of thought processes.
   2. Anxiety.
   3. Impaired cognitive functioning.
   4. Powerlessness.

Answer: 4

Rationale: When a client has feelings of not being able to control a situation or the outcome of their illness, they experience feelings of powerlessness. Impaired thought processes, anxiety, and impaired cognitive functioning are not related to this situation.

Client Need: Psychosocial Integrity

53.   A pediatric client with leukemia is admitted to your unit. The child is to receive chemotherapy. The nurse reviewing the child's laboratory results notes that the platelet count is dangerously low. Based on this platelet count, which of the following is the nurse's priority intervention?

1. Place the child in protective isolation.
2. Place the child on bleeding precautions.
3. Place the child on contact isolation.
4. Place the child on respiratory isolation.

Answer: 2

Rationale: When the platelet count is dangerously low, clients are at risk for bleeding. The nurse's responsibility is then to initiate bleeding precautions. Placing the child in protective isolation is appropriate for a dangerously low white blood cell count. Contact precautions and respiratory isolation are not necessary in this situation.

Client Need: Physiological Integrity

54.   A nurse enters a client's room to find the client having a seizure. The nurse notes that the client's body becomes rigid, alternating with periods of relaxation. The nurse correctly documents that the client has experienced what type of seizure?

_____

Answer: Generalized tonic clonic seizure

Rationale: Generalized tonic clonic seizures occur bilaterally. The client experiences contractions alternating with periods of relaxation.

Client Need: Physiological Integrity

55.   A nurse is to administer an iron injection to an adult client. The nurse knows that to administer this medication it is recommended to use which technique?

_____

Answer: Z track

Rationale: The correct technique for administering iron preparation is using the Z track technique while injecting the medication deep into the gluteal muscle.

Client Need: Physiological Integrity

56.   A female client with a suspected bladder infection is asked to provide the nurse with a midstream urine sample. Which of the following statements, if made by the client, indicates an understanding of the procedure?

1. "Douching before I collect the urine specimen is beneficial."
2. "I will need to cleanse my perineal area from front to back."
3. "It is important that I collect every drop of urine."
4. "I will collect my urine tonight before going to bed and keep it refrigerated overnight."

Answer: 2

> Did you use 3 Bs and 1 G for this teaching question?

Rationale: Part of the procedure for collecting a midstream urine sample is to teach the client to cleanse the perineum from front to back. Douching is not part of the collection procedure. The client is instructed to allow some urine to pass before collecting the specimen. The urine must be taken to the lab as soon as it is collected.

Client Need: Physiological Integrity

57.   A pediatric client in a sickle cell crisis comes to the hospital with his mother. When assessing the client, the nurse knows that which of the following is the most frequent sign and symptom of this disorder?

   1. Tachycardia.
   2. Bradycardia.
   3. Pain.
   4. Constipation.

Answer: 3

Rationale: The most common sign and symptom a client will experience in a sickle cell crisis is acute pain. Answers 1, 2, and 4 are not associated with a sickle cell crisis.

> Did you know the answer or use step 5 to answer this question?

Client Need: Physiological Integrity

58.   A client is receiving a unit of packed red blood cells. The nurse monitoring the client notices that the client's skin is flushed and the client is complaining of a backache. The nurse suspects the client is having a transfusion reaction. The nurse's next priority action is to do which of the following?

   1. Discontinue the blood and the intravenous line.
   2. Discontinue the blood and infuse 5% dextrose in water.
   3. Continue transfusing the blood and monitor the client closely.
   4. Discontinue the blood and infuse normal saline solution.

Answer: 4

Rationale: A nurse who suspects a client is having a blood transfusion reaction should immediately stop the infusion and begin administering a solution of normal saline. The client's intravenous line should not be interrupted. The nurse should not infuse dextrose 5% in water or continue the blood transfusion.

Client Need: Physiological Integrity

59.   An adolescent with asthma is taking albuterol (Ventolin) by inhaler and has had difficulty with coughing up secretions. The nurse teaches the adolescent which of the following to best help clear bronchial secretions?

   1.   "Take an extra dose of the inhaler every morning."
   2.   "Increase fluid intake to 2000 to 3000 ml a day."
   3.   "Participate in an extracurricular activity each day."
   4.   "Tell your parents to put a dehumidifier in your bedroom."

Answer: 2

Rationale: It is important to increase fluid intake to 2000 to 3000 ml a day to make secretions less viscous. It is not appropriate to have the adolescent take an extra dose of the inhaler. Participating in extracurricular activities and using a dehumidifier will not help the adolescent to cough up secretions.

Client Need: Health Promotion and Maintenance

60.   A young adult is being discharged from the emergency room after being fitted for crutches to assist him in ambulation. The nurse knows the client needs further teaching when the client states which of the following?

   1.   "I will keep spare crutch tips handy."
   2.   "I will bear the weight of my body on my hands."
   3.   "I will inspect my crutches every day for signs of wear."
   4.   "I have a set of spare crutches in my basement I can use if needed."

Answer: 4

Rationale: Clients using crutches need to inspect them frequently and keep spare parts handy. It is important that the client bear the weight of his body on his hands and not the axilla. The client should not use a set of crutches he found in his basement that belonged to someone else. He should be encouraged to use crutches that have been fitted especially for him.

Client Need: Health Promotion and Maintenance

61.   A client visits his primary care physician and complains of experiencing periods of sadness. The physician orders Prozac. The nurse providing teaching to the client regarding the administration of Prozac knows the client has understood the teaching when the client states which of the following?

   1. "I will take this medicine at bedtime."
   2. "I will take this medicine after dinner."
   3. "I will take this medicine with an antacid to prevent stomach irritation."
   4. "I will take this medicine first thing in the morning."

   Answer: 4

   Rationale: Prozac is correctly administered when it is taken first thing in the morning. Answers 1, 2, and 3 are incorrect.

   Client Need: Health Promotion and Maintenance

   Did you try using "true" and "false" with this question?

62.   A client who has had a total knee replacement is being discharged to a rehabilitation center. The nurse completes discharge teaching and knows that the client needs further instructions when the client states which of the following?

   1. "Any signs of bleeding in my gums or in my stool should be reported to my doctor."
   2. "I need to tell the rehabilitation caregivers about the metal implant."
   3. "I will call my physician if I develop a fever, redness, or increased pain in my knee."
   4. "I know that the shape of my knee will change as I heal."

   Answer: 4

   Rationale: After a total knee replacement, the client should be instructed to report any signs of bleeding and infection. It is important for the client to know he must tell future caregivers about his metal implant. It is not an expected outcome for the shape of the client's knee to change post-operatively. This should be reported to the surgeon immediately.

Client Need: Health Promotion and Maintenance

---

63. A client is prescribed Colace. The nurse teaches the client to monitor for which of the following intended effects of this medication?

1. Decreased bowel movements.
2. Regular bowel movements.
3. Decrease in fatty stools.
4. Decrease in diarrhea.

Answer: 2

Rationale: Colace is a stool softener that promotes absorption of water into the stool. The intended outcome is to produce stool that is softer in consistency and easier for the client to pass.

Client Need: Health Promotion and Maintenance

---

64. A client is suspected of having a diagnosis of pernicious anemia. The nurse anticipates the physician to order which diagnostic test?

_____

Answer: Schilling test

Rationale: Schilling test is used to determine the cause of vitamin B_{12} deficiency, which leads to pernicious anemia.

Client Need: Physiological Integrity

65. A child is diagnosed with attention deficit disorder and is prescribed Ritalin. The nurse providing instructions to the mother regarding the administration of this medication correctly tells the mother to administer the medication at which of the following times?

  1. At bedtime.
  2. First thing in the morning.
  3. At lunchtime.
  4. At dinnertime.

Answer: 3

Rationale: Ritalin should not be taken by children after 1 p.m. The stimulating effect of the drug may keep the child awake at bedtime. Answers 1, 2, and 4 are incorrect.

> Step 5 can help here if the facts are unknown.

Client Need: Health Promotion and Maintenance

66. A client is taking aluminum hydroxide (Amphojel) as needed for periods of heartburn. The client tells the nurse that the heartburn is relieved. What common side effect will the nurse anticipate the client may complain about while taking the medication?

  1. Constipation.
  2. Sleepiness.
  3. Muscle spasm.
  4. Lightheadedness.

Answer: 1

Rationale: Aluminum hydroxide has been known to cause constipation in many clients. Answers 2, 3, and 4 are not appropriate here.

Client Need: Health Promotion and Maintenance

67.   A 62-year-old woman is admitted to the hospital for abdominal surgery. The nurse is preparing to implement a preoperative teaching plan and will focus primarily on which of the following?

1. What the client knows about the surgery.
2. The client's usual coping mechanisms.
3. The client's current home environment.
4. Family members who will help care for the client at discharge.

Answer: 1

Rationale: The first step in preoperative teaching is to find out what the client knows about the surgical procedure. This allows the nurse to implement necessary teaching and correct any misinformation. Discussing the clients coping mechanisms, home environment, and family members who can help with the care of the clients at discharge time are important but not the priority at this time.

Did you remember that nurses Assess Before Caring?

Client Need: Psychosocial Integrity

68.   A client has been diagnosed with Bell's palsy. The nurse assesses the client and expects to see which of the following **most** common signs and symptoms of this disorder?

1. Difficulty with speech and one-sided facial drooping.
2. Dilated pupils and an elevated eyelid.
3. Paralysis of the eye and loss of hearing in the ear on the affected side.
4. Twitching on one side of the face and excess nasal discharge.

Answer: 1

Rationale: One-sided facial paralysis and speech difficulties are characteristics seen in clients with Bell's palsy. Answers 2, 3, and 4 are incorrect.

Client Need: Physiological Integrity

69.   A client falls off his bike and suffers a fractured tibia. He comes to the clinic, and the x-ray shows that the bone is completely fractured along the shaft with small splintered pieces around it. The nurse knows that this client's fracture is known as _____.

> **Answer:** Comminuted
>
> **Rationale:** A comminuted fracture is a complete fracture of a bone with splintering into small fragments.
>
> **Client Need:** Physiological Integrity

70.   A prenatal client comes to the clinic at 39 weeks gestation. The nurse notes the client has extensive edema of the lower extremities. The nurse assesses the level of edema by pressing an index finger against the shin and holding the pressure for 2 to 3 seconds. The nurse notes that the indentation is approximately ¼" deep. The nurse correctly documents that the client has which level of pitting edema?

> 1. 4+ edema.
> 2. 3+ edema.
> 3. 2+ edema.
> 4. 1+ edema.
>
> **Answer:** 3
>
> **Rationale:** 2+ edema leaves an indentation of approximately ¼". 4+ edema leaves an indentation of approximately 1 inch. 3+ edema leaves an indentation of approximately ½". 1+ edema leaves a slight indentation.
>
> **Step 5 works here if the facts are unknown.**
>
> **Client Need:** Health Promotion and Maintenance

71.   A client is to have an abdominal paracentesis. After signing a procedural consent, the nurse assists the client to assume which of the following correct positions?

   1. High Fowler's.
   2. Semi-Fowler's.
   3. Low Fowler's.
   4. Supine.

   Answer: 1

   Rationale: For an abdominal paracentesis the nurse should position the client in a high Fowler's position. This allows for pooling of the fluid. The other positions are inappropriate for this procedure.

   Client Need: Physiological Integrity

72.   A client has sustained a fracture to the left lower arm. Which of the following signs and symptoms if observed by the nurse are consistent with impaired venous return on the affected arm?

   1. A bounding distal pulse.
   2. Acute pain.
   3. Pallor of the surrounding skin.
   4. Increasing edema.

   Answer: 4

   Rationale: Increasing edema is a characteristic sign and symptom of impaired venous return. In a client with an arm fracture, increasing edema can be prevented by elevating the limb.

   Client Need: Physiological Integrity

73.   A new mother on her second day postpartum complains of nipple soreness and cracking. The nurse recommends that the mother do which of the following to help lessen discomfort during breastfeeding? Select all that apply.

1. Apply breastmilk to nipples after each feeding and allow to air dry.
2. Alternate breasts at the beginning of each feeding.
3. Let the baby sleep for long periods so breasts can heal.
4. Give the baby some formula at the beginning of each feeding to decrease the infant's hunger.
5. Change the infant's position on the nipples with each feeding.

Answers: 1, 2, and 5

Rationale: It is important for the mother to alternate breasts at the beginning of each feeding. Applying breast milk to the nipples after each feeding and allowing to air dry helps with healing cracked nipples. Changing the infant's position on the nipples with each feeding is helpful in decreasing stress on the nipples. It is not a good idea to allow the baby to sleep for prolonged periods because the baby may become overly hungry and eat aggressively. It is not recommended to give the infant a bottle at the beginning of each feeding.

Client Need: Physiological Integrity

74. A client comes to the outpatient clinic after having sprained his right ankle. When preparing to discharge the client home, the nurse completes discharge instructions. The nurse determines that teaching has been effective when the client states which of the following?

1. "I will apply ice to my ankle for 20 minutes every hour."
2. "I will rewrap my ankle in the ace bandage starting from the knee down."
3. "I will walk on my ankle for 20 minutes every hour."
4. "I will keep a heating pad on my ankle while I sleep tonight."

Answer: 1

Rationale: Acceptable treatment for a sprained ankle is the application of ice for 20 minutes out of every hour for the first 24 hours. Ace bandages should be applied when needed and wrapped toward the heart. The client should avoid walking on the ankle for the next few days. The application of heat is inappropriate.

Client Need: Physiological Integrity

75. As part of an annual physical a client is to have a chest x-ray. The nurse correctly provides the client with which instruction before the procedure?

1. Remove all metal necklaces.
2. Take several shallow breaths during the x-ray procedure.
3. Remain NPO the morning of the test.
4. Expect minor discomfort associated with the procedure.

Answer: 1

Rationale: All metal jewelry should be removed in the area to be x-rayed. The client will be asked to hold his or her breath during the x-ray procedure. There is no reason to fast the morning of the test. There is no discomfort associated with a chest x-ray.

> **Ah-ha! Did you remember to take some deep breaths and stretch?**

Client Need: Physiological Integrity

76. A client newly diagnosed with Bell's palsy is distressed about the change in her facial appearance. The nurse teaches the client about the following characteristics of Bell's palsy to help the client cope with the disorder:

1. Remind the client that the symptoms will completely go away after surgery.
2. Tell the client the facial changes will resolve with medication.
3. Instruct the client that Bell's palsy is similar to a stroke.
4. Teach the client that Bell's palsy is not caused by a stroke, and many clients recover after 3 to 5 weeks.

Answer: 4

Rationale: Clients with Bell's palsy need reassurance that they have not had a stroke and that there is a good chance their symptoms will disappear spontaneously in a little over a month's time. Clients with Bell's palsy do not require surgery.

> Did you use step 4 to answer this question?

Client Need: Psychosocial Integrity

---

77. A young male client diagnosed with myasthenia gravis comes to the emergency department in crisis. The nurse knows that the occurrence of a crisis for this client most likely has been precipitated by which of the following factors?

    1. The client is not taking the prescribed medication.
    2. The client is taking too much prescribed medication.
    3. The client is not getting enough sleep.
    4. The client is ingesting an excess amount of food.

Answer: 1

Rationale: Clients with myasthenia gravis in crisis are usually not taking the prescribed medication or are taking too little of the prescribed medication. Taking an excess amount of medication is associated with a cholinergic crisis. A change in the client's diet and sleeping habits is not associated with a crisis.

Client Need: Physiological Integrity

---

78. A client is to receive 5000 units of heparin intrafat. Which of the following procedures is correct for the nurse to follow in administering this medication?

    1. Inject the medication above the level of the umbilicus.
    2. Inject the medication in the deltoid muscle.
    3. Inject the medication in the vastus lateralis.
    4. Massage the injection site after administration of the medication.

Answer: 1

Rationale: Heparin is injected into the abdominal fat layer 1 to 2 inches above the umbilicus. The injection site is not massaged.

Client Need: Physiological Integrity

---

79.   A newly delivered newborn is brought to the nursery. The nurse performs an admission assessment, which includes vital signs. Which of the following findings indicates a normal newborn respiratory rate?

1.   22 breaths per minute.
2.   48 breaths per minute.
3.   100 breaths per minute.
4.   110 breaths per minute.

Answer: 2

Rationale: The normal respiratory rate for a newborn ranges between 30 and 60 breaths per minute. A rate of 22 breaths per minute is bradypnea. Answers 3 and 4 are considered tachypnea.

Client Need: Physiological Integrity

---

80.   A client returns from the postanesthesia care unit. The following morning the client complains of gas pains and requests medication. The nurse reviews the physician's medication order, expecting to find which of the following medications?

1.   Motrin.
2.   Mylicon.
3.   Milk of magnesium.
4.   Demerol.

Answer: 2

Rationale: Mylicon is used postoperatively for clients experiencing gas pains. It is an antiflatulent that works directly on the gastrointestinal tract. The other medications are not used to relieve gas pains.

Client Need: Physiological Integrity

---

81. A client is being discharged from the hospital after recovering from carbon monoxide poisoning from a suicide attempt. The nurse anticipates the physician will order a consultation for which of the following health services?

1. Cardiac rehabilitation.
2. Occupational therapy.
3. Hematologist.
4. Psychiatrist.

Answer: 4

Rationale: A client recovering from carbon monoxide poisoning as a result of a suicide attempt should have a mental health consultation done as soon as possible. Cardiac rehabilitation, occupational therapy, and hematology are not indicated at this time.

Ah-ha! Time to breathe deep and stretch.

Client Need: Psychosocial Integrity

---

82. A post-term small for gestational age newborn is admitted to the newborn nursery. The nursery nurse develops a plan of care for the infant and includes which of the following nursing interventions as *priority*?

1. Monitor intake and output.
2. Monitor bilirubin level.
3. Monitor blood glucose levels.
4. Monitor hemoglobin and hematocrit levels.

Answer: 3

Rationale: The most common metabolic complication associated with small for gestational age neonates is hypoglycemia. Monitoring urinary output, bilirubin levels, and hemoglobin and hematocrit are important but are not priority in the situation.

Did step 5 help you with this question?

Client Need: Physiological Integrity

---

83.   A client is receiving pancreatic enzymes as a digestive aid. The client should be instructed to expect which of the following gastrointestinal changes?

1. Increased fat in stools.
2. Decreased black tarry stools.
3. Increased watery stools.
4. Decreased fat in stools.

Answer: 4

Rationale: Clients receiving pancreatic enzymes as a digestive aid should expect to have a reduction of fat in their stools. Black tarry stools and watery stools are not associated with pancreatic enzyme use.

Client Need: Physiological Integrity

---

84.   A client has just returned to the unit after a mastectomy. The nurse assigned to the client assists her in doing which of the following exercises during the first postoperative 24 hours? Select all that apply.

1. Flexion and extension of the fingers.
2. Flexion and extension of the hands.
3. Flexion and extension of the elbow.
4. Rotation of the shoulder.
5. Wall climbing exercise.

Answers: 1, 2, and 3

Rationale: During the first postoperative 24 hours the client with a mastectomy should be encouraged to flex and extend the fingers, the hands, and the elbows on the affected side. Rotation of the shoulder and wall climbing exercises are not done during this period.

Client Need: Physiological Integrity

---

85.   A nurse is preparing to teach a client how to draw regular insulin and NPH insulin in the same syringe. Which instructions would the nurse tell the client to follow in preparing to self-inject a syringe of mixed insulin?

1. Draw up the NPH insulin into the syringe first.
2. Inject air into the regular insulin first.
3. Shake the NPH insulin until it is well mixed.
4. Rotate the regular insulin bottle in the palms of the hands before mixing.

Answer: 4

Rationale: Rotating the regular insulin bottle in the palms of the hands before mixing is recommended. When mixing regular and NPH insulin, regular insulin is drawn into the syringe first. The nurse injects air into the NPH insulin and then into the regular insulin. It is never recommended to shake insulin.

> Did step 4 help with this question?

Client Need: Health Promotion and Maintenance

---

86.   A client tells the nurse she took a dose of Dramamine before coming to the health care clinic. The nurse determines that the medication is effective if the client obtains relief of which of the following signs and symptoms?

1. Nausea and vomiting.
2. Tinnitus.
3. Headache.
4. Fever.

Answer: 1

Rationale: Dramamine is used to treat and prevent the signs and symptoms of nausea and vomiting often associated with dizziness, vertigo, and motion sickness. Answers 2, 3, and 4 are incorrect.

Client Need: Physiological Integrity

---

87. A client has been taking Prilosec for the past 4 weeks. The nurse determines that the medication has been effective if the client reports relief from which of the following signs and symptoms?

1. Constipation.
2. Diarrhea.
3. Flatulence.
4. Acid indigestion.

Answer: 4

Rationale: Prilosec is a medication used for the relief of gastric irritation often referred to as heartburn by clients. This medication does not affect the other symptoms listed.

Client Need: Physiological Integrity

---

88. A client admitted to a psychiatric health care unit is prescribed Antabuse by his physician. The nurse is completing the admission assessment and includes instructions regarding the use of this medication. Which of the following information is **most** important for the nurse to obtain before beginning the administration of Antabuse?

1. The client's history of thyroid disease.
2. The client's history of hypertension.
3. When the client last drank alcohol.
4. When the client last ate a full meal.

Answer: 3

Rationale: Antabuse is used in the treatment of chronic alcoholism in clients who want to remain sober. It is important that the clients on Antabuse abstain from drinking alcohol for at least 12 hours before beginning the medication. The client's past medical history is important but not to the priority at this time.

Client Need: Physiological Integrity

89.   A client diagnosed with type 2 diabetes has been well controlled while taking oral diabetic medications. The client reports a morning fasting blood glucose level of greater than 180 mg/dl for the past week. On further assessment, the nurse determines that which of the following client medications may be a contributing factor in elevating the client's morning blood glucose level?

1. Zantac.
2. Keflex.
3. Prednisone.
4. Tagamet.

Answer: 3

Rationale: Corticosteroids, such as prednisone, may decrease the effects of oral diabetic medications and cause hyperglycemia. Answers 1, 2, and 4 are not associated with hyperglycemia.

Did you use step 5 to answer this question?

Client Need: Physiological Integrity

90.   A postpartum nurse receives a client who has just delivered a normal healthy neonate. The nurse notes on the client's chart that Methergine was administered intramuscularly in the delivery room. The nurse knows that the purpose of this medication is to do which of the following?

1. Decrease afterpains.
2. Raise the client's blood pressure.
3. Prevent postpartum hemorrhage.
4. Encourage the flow of lochia rubra.

Answer: 3

Rationale: The purpose of this medication is to cause uterine contractions in controlling postpartum bleeding. Initially, Methergine is administered intramuscularly and then by mouth if further dosing is required.

Remembering Airway, Breathing, and Circulation or using step 5 works for this question.

Client Need: Physiological Integrity

91. A newly admitted male client has just received a dose of diazepam (Valium). The nurse administering the medication would take which of the following important nursing actions before exiting the client's room?

1. Turn off the overhead lights.
2. Turn off the bell on the client's telephone.
3. Put up the side rails on the client's bed.
4. Turn off the client's television.

Answer: 3

Rationale: Valium or diazepam is used as a sedative/hypnotic medication. The nurse should institute safety measures before leaving the client's room to include putting up the client's side rails, placing the bed in the lowest position, and placing the client's call bell within reach.

Did you remember "safety" as the priority for this client?

Client Need: Safe Effective Care Environment

92.   A client diagnosed with angina pectoris is experiencing chest pain and has taken three sublingual nitroglycerin tablets. The client reports relief from the chest pain but is now complaining of a headache. The nurse correctly determines that this symptom **most likely** represents which of the following?

1.   An allergy to the nitroglycerin.
2.   An expected side effect of the medication.
3.   An indication that the client is developing a tolerance to the medication.
4.   An indication of a need to change the client's medication.

Answer: 2

Rationale: Headache is a frequent side effect for clients using nitroglycerin. The resulting vasodilation causes an increased blood flow to the head. Answers 1, 3, and 4 are incorrect.

Client Need: Physiological Integrity

93.   A postoperative client is diagnosed with anemia secondary to excess blood loss during a recent surgery. The nurse interprets which of the following client complaints as most likely associated with the client's anemia?

1.   Fatigue.
2.   Tachypnea.
3.   Bradycardia.
4.   Muscle cramps.

Answer: 1

Rationale: A postoperative client who develops anemia secondary to excessive blood loss during surgery will likely complain of fatigue. This is due to the decreased ability of the body to carry oxygen to vital tissues and organs. The client is likely to experience tachycardia and shortness of breath. Muscle cramps are not associated with anemia.

Client Need: Physiological Integrity

94. A client diagnosed with angina pectoris has begun using nitroglycerin transdermal patches. The nurse provides directions for the client regarding proper use of this medication system and instructs the client to do which of the following?

1. Apply a new transdermal patch once a week.
2. Apply the transdermal patch every morning and leave in place for 12 hours.
3. Apply the transdermal patch to skin located below the level of the waist.
4. Wait 24 hours to apply a new patch if the existing patch falls off.

Answer: 2

Rationale: A client using a nitroglycerin transdermal patch should apply the patch every morning after showering and leave in place for a minimum of 12 hours. A client should not leave a patch on for 7 days. The patch is applied to skin located closest to the chest area.

Client Need: Health Promotion and Maintenance

95. A client with a long-standing history of chronic ulcerative colitis is diagnosed with anemia. The nurse understands that which of the following factors is **most** likely responsible for the client's anemia?

1. Decreased iron in the client's diet.
2. Intestinal malabsorption syndrome.
3. Long-standing blood loss.
4. Intestinal parasites.

Answer: 3

Rationale: A client with long-standing ulcerative colitis is most likely anemic due to chronic blood loss in small amounts that occurs over time. These clients often report bloody stools and are therefore at

> Did you notice the use of the phrase "long-standing" in the question *and* the correct answer?

increased risk for developing anemia. Answers 1, 2, and 4 do not apply in this situation.

Client Need: Physiological Integrity

---

96. A client is scheduled for a bone marrow aspiration. He asks the nurse about possible sites that could be used for the procedure. The nurse tells the client that in addition to the iliac crest, the **most** common site for bone marrow aspiration is which of the following?

1. The femur.
2. The humerus.
3. The sternum.
4. The ribs.

Answer: 3

Rationale: The most common sites for bone marrow aspiration in the adult include the iliac crest and the sternum. The femur, the humerus, and the ribs are not used for bone marrow aspiration.

> Did step 5 help with this question?

Client Need: Physiological Integrity

---

97. A postoperative client has a hemoglobin level that is low. The physician orders the client to be transfused with one unit of packed red blood cells. In addition, the physician prescribes a dose of Benadryl to be administered to the client before administration of the blood transfusion. The nurse determines that this medication has been prescribed to do which of the following?

1. Prevent the formation of urticaria.
2. Prevent the client from developing a fever.
3. Prevent the client from fluid overload.
4. Prevent the formation of erythroblasts.

Answer: 1

Rationale: Benadryl is an antihistamine given to prevent the formation of urticaria associated with a transfusion reaction. Answers 2, 3, and 4 are incorrect.

Client Need: Physiological Integrity

98.   A client diagnosed with myasthenia gravis tells the nurse that he continues to experience fatigue. The nurse determines that the client's medication regimen needs adjusting when the client tells the nurse he experiences fatigue at which of the following times?

1. Before meals.
2. Waking up in the morning.
3. After exercising.
4. After meals.

Answer: 3

Rationale: The client with myasthenia gravis commonly experiences fatigue after periods of exercise and most often at bedtime. The nurse would suggest to the client to arrange activities to conserve energy and muscle strength. The client should continue to take his medication as prescribed by his physician.

Client Need: Physiological Integrity

99.   The nursing instructor is teaching a class of students on the proper care of clients diagnosed with intracranial aneurysms and who are placed on aneurysm precautions. The nursing instructor knows teaching was effective when a student nurse states that which of the following interventions supports aneurysm precautions?

1. Clients with aneurysms develop photosensitivity and need to be kept in isolation.
2. It is important to reduce environmental stimuli to prevent rupture of the aneurysm.
3. Decreased sensory stimulation promotes healing of the aneurysm.
4. It is necessary to limit the client's hallway ambulation to once a shift.

Answer: 2

Rationale: Clients on aneurysm precautions are at risk for bleeding or rupture of the aneurysm. It is important to minimize environmental stimuli and to avoid increasing intracranial pressure. The client does not need to be kept in isolation. Reducing sensory stimulation does not promote healing of the aneurysm.

Client Need: Psychosocial Integrity

100. A client diagnosed with acute renal failure has an elevated blood urea nitrogen (BUN) blood level. Which of the following signs and symptoms will the nurse anticipate the client to experience due to the elevated BUN level?

1. Forgetfulness.
2. Euphoria.
3. Insomnia.
4. Ambivalence.

Answer: 1

Rationale: Clients diagnosed with acute renal failure with elevated BUN levels have difficulty remembering information and instructions. Euphoria, insomnia, and ambivalence are not associated with an elevated BUN level.

Client Need: Psychosocial Integrity

101. The nurse knows that caring for postoperative clients includes maintaining the client's safety. In planning client care postoperatively, the nurse includes all the following interventions **except**

    1. Placing the call bell within the client's reach.

    2. Answering the call bell promptly.

    3. Leaving the side rails in the low position.

    4. Keeping a night light on in the bathroom.

Answer: 3

Rationale: Maintaining client safety is a priority nursing goal. Keeping the client's call bell within reach, answering the call bell promptly, and keeping a night light on in the bathroom are all measures to help ensure client safety. Leaving the side rails in the low position for the postoperative client is contraindicated.

> Did you notice the **bold** word in the question?

Client Need: Safe Effective Care Environment

102. A 43-year-old obese woman has been working with the nurse on a weight reduction program. Which of the following statements, if made by the client, indicates to the nurse that additional teaching is needed?

    1. "I wish some of my high school friends could see me now."

    2. "Sometimes it's hard to find foods that I can eat that taste good and fill me up."

    3. "My husband tells me I look sexy again."

    4. "It's unfortunate that I can no longer go out to lunch with my friends."

Answer: 4

Rationale: If the client believes she cannot go out to lunch with her friends she may not make appropriate choices for her food exchanges. A sense of not being able to take part in social activities can leave the obese client feeling isolated and make it more difficult for the client to maintain the diet. Responses 1, 2, and 3 are not indicated here.

Client Need: Health Promotion and Maintenance

---

103. A client diagnosed with rheumatoid arthritis has Motrin 300 mg orally ordered for pain. The client asks the nurse about the amount of medication prescribed by the physician. The nurse's response to the client is based on the understanding that the prescribed dosage is which of the following?

1. The normal adult dose.
2. Less than the normal adult dose.
3. Greater than the normal adult dose.
4. Indicative of the client's diagnosis.

Answer: 1

Rationale: The normal adult dose for Motrin is 300 to 800 mg three to four times daily. Therefore answers 2, 3, and 4 are incorrect.

Client Need: Physiological Integrity

---

104. A mother calls the pediatrician's office to report that her child has a bloody nose. The nurse offers the mother the following instructions to assist in stopping the bleeding.

1. Place the child in a sitting position with the head tilted back.
2. Pinch the nostrils for no longer than 5 minutes and recheck for bleeding.
3. Place the child in a supine position with a pillow under the back.
4. Have the child sit with the head tilted forward and hold pressure on the nose for 10 minutes.

Answer: 4

Rationale: It is best for a child with a bloody nose (epistaxis) to be positioned in an erect manner with the head tilted forward to prevent blood from running down the pharynx. The soft part of the nose should be pinched for at least 10 minutes and then the child should be checked for further bleeding.

> **Did you notice number 4 was the most comprehensive answer? It gives the mother more direction than the other answers.**

Client Need: Physiological Integrity

---

105. A child is admitted to the pediatric unit after falling from a piece of equipment at the local playground. The child has sustained a head injury. The nurse knows that it is most important to include which of the following interventions in the care of this child?

1. Keep the child lying flat in bed.
2. Keep the child NPO.
3. Keep the child awake as much as possible.
4. Complete neurological assessments every morning.

Answer: 3

Rationale: A child with a head injury should be kept in a high Fowler's position to decrease intracranial pressure. The child should be encouraged to drink fluids, and neurological assessments should be done more frequently. Keeping the child awake as much as possible will assist the nurse in determining if cerebral edema is occurring.

Client Need: Physiological Integrity

---

106. A nursing instructor is teaching a student how to care for a client with a closed chest drainage system. The nursing instructor determines that the student has understood the teaching when the student states which of the following is evidence of lung expansion?

1. "The client's oxygen saturation is 95%."
2. "Fluctuations in the water seal chamber have ceased."
3. "The client no longer complains of pleuritic chest pain."
4. "The client refuses to wear the oxygen cannula."

Answer: 2

Rationale: A classic indication that lung expansion has occurred is when fluctuation in the water seal drainage has ceased. An oxygen saturation rate of 95%, decreased complaints of pleuritic chest pain, and refusal to wear oxygen are not indicators of lung expansion.

Client Need: Physiological Integrity

107.   A delivery room nurse is assessing a client who has just had a normal spontaneous vaginal delivery of a healthy baby boy. The nurse assesses the uterine fundus and anticipates noting that the fundus is located at what position on the client's abdomen?

1. At the level of the umbilicus.
2. Three finger breadths above the umbilicus.
3. One finger breadth above the symphysis pubis.
4. To the right of the umbilicus.

Answer: 1

Rationale: The uterine fundus is typically found at or just below the level of the umbilicus immediately after delivery. A fundus that is three finger breadths above the umbilicus may indicate blood clots in the uterus. The fundus would not be found just above the symphysis pubis. A uterine fundus that is deviated to the right of the umbilicus indicates a full bladder.

Client Need: Physiological Integrity

108. A nursing instructor is testing nursing students on suicide and suicide plans. The nursing instructor determines that a nursing student understands the concepts associated with suicide and suicide plans if the student includes which of the following in his or her answer?

    1. Suicidal tendencies are seen in families, so there is little we can do to prevent it.
    2. People who attempt suicide are only looking for attention.
    3. Often, individuals who succeed in committing suicide have told others of their suicide plans.
    4. Only people diagnosed with schizophrenia commit suicide.

Answer: 3

Rationale: Very often, individuals who succeed in committing suicide have discussed their suicide plans with others. There is much health care providers can do to prevent suicide. People who attempt suicide are not only looking for attention. People who are not schizophrenic also attempt suicide.

> **Did you notice the word "only" in options 2 and 4? It should have been a clue to discard both answers.**

Client Need: Psychosocial Integrity

109. A woman in the third trimester of pregnancy is attending childbirth classes. The instructor teaches the woman how to perform Kegel exercises and the purpose for the exercises. Which statement, if made by the pregnant woman, indicates to the nurse that teaching was successful?

    1. "These exercises will help reduce swelling of my feet."
    2. "These exercises will help me push when the time comes."
    3. "These exercises will help lessen my back aches."
    4. "These exercises will prevent further stretch marks."

Answer: 2

Rationale: Kegel exercises help to strengthen perineal muscles, which help the mother to push in the second stage of labor. The exercises do not reduce backaches, lessen stretch marks, or reduce ankle edema.

Client Need: Health Promotion and Maintenance

Did you use a G and 3 Bs? Remember, teaching was effective in this question. Responses 1, 3, and 4 are incorrect information. Answer 2 is accurate information.

110. A client comes to the emergency department with a fractured leg. The client's fracture is to be reduced in the casting room. What is the nurse's **priority** intervention?

1. Have the anesthesiologist see the client.
2. Have the client sign an informed consent for treatment.
3. Notify the surgeon on call.
4. Administer a narcotic analgesic for pain.

Answer: 2

Rationale: Before a casting procedure can be completed, the client must sign an informed consent for treatment. There is no need to notify an anesthesiologist or a surgeon. Narcotic analgesics would not be administered until the consent is signed.

Client Need: Physiological Integrity

111. A client newly diagnosed with Bell's palsy sees his physician. The nurse anticipates the physician writing an order for which medication commonly used in the treatment of Bell's palsy?

_____

Answer: Prednisone

Rationale: Bell's palsy is usually treated successfully with prednisone. This medication helps to reduce inflammation and edema, thus allowing normal circulation to return to the nerves involved.

Client Need: Physiological Integrity

112. A postoperative client suddenly develops difficulty breathing in the postanesthesia care unit. The client is placed on mechanical ventilation and brought to the intensive care unit. The client becomes visibly upset and anxious. What is the nurse's **best action** to alleviate the client's anxiety?

1. Assign a nursing assistant to stay with the client.
2. Request a family member stay with the client.
3. Medicate the client with a narcotic analgesic.
4. Stay with the client and provide verbal reassurance.

Answer: 4

Rationale: The nurse should remain with the client and provide the client with verbal reassurance. It is not appropriate to ask a family member to take on the responsibility of staying with the client. Asking a nursing assistant to sit with the client and administering a dose of narcotic analgesic medication are not appropriate at this time.

Did you remember to be accountable for what is clearly a nursing responsibility?

Client Need: Psychosocial Integrity

1.   A nurse caring for a preterm infant in an incubator knows the maximum oxygen concentration safe to be administered is _____.

> **Answer:** 40%
>
> **Rationale:** Oxygen concentrations greater than 40% can cause retinal damage and visual impairment.
>
> **Client Need:** Health Promotion and Maintenance

2.   A client with second- and third-degree burns returns from the operating room after a skin grafting procedure. The nurse correctly expects to assess all the following **except**

> 1.   A splint on the affected joint.
> 2.   A wet to dry dressing on the graft.
> 3.   A sterile dressing on the donor site.
> 4.   A pressure dressing on the surgical site.

> **Answer:** 2
>
> **Rationale:** A wet to dry dressing is used to debride dead tissue. A graft site has a pressure dressing and splint to immobilize the new tissue to assist in the establishment of a blood supply. The donor site has a plain sterile dressing.
>
> | Did you notice the word "except"? It is important to know exactly what the question is asking you. |
>
> **Client Need:** Physiological Integrity

3.   The client has intravenous solution of the D5 and 0.45 normal saline started at 8 a.m. The physician orders a total of 3000 ml of the same intravenous fluid over the next 24 hours. At what time should the nurse prepare to hang the second intravenous bag?

_____

Answer: 4 p.m.

Rationale: Each bag infuses for 8 hours. The next bag is due to be hung at 4 p.m. The third bag will be hung at 12 midnight.

Client Need: Physiological Integrity

> **Did you remember to label your answer with "p.m."? The label was not specified in the question.**

4. The absence or the suppression of menses is known as _____.

Answer: Amenorrhea

Rationale: Amenorrhea is only normal before puberty, after menopause, and during pregnancy.

Client Need: Physiological Integrity

5. A 78-year-old recently widowed man is unable to drive himself to the store and is afraid to cook on the stove. The nurse should recommend which of the following community resources?

1. Hospice care.
2. Meals on Wheels.
3. Visiting nurse services.
4. The American Association of Retired Persons.

Answer: 2

Rationale: Meals on Wheels is a program that provides nutritious food to needy clients once a day in their homes and checks on the client's well-being. Hospice care is for terminally ill clients. Visiting nurse services provide skilled nursing care in the client's home. The American Association of Retired Persons (AARP) is a national organization for people over 50 years old. They do not provide health care.

Client Need: Safe Effective Care Environment

6.   The nurse is teaching the parents of a 2-year-old in a hip spica cast how to feed their toddler safely. The nurse understands that teaching has been effective when the parents state which of the following?

1. "There are special feeding tables to help us."
2. "Laying our son flat will help him eat more."
3. "I will feed my son while my husband holds him on his lap."
4. "Keeping our son sitting upright is important."

Answer: 1

Rationale: There are special feeding trays and tables available and specially modified highchairs the parents can utilize. The child should never be flat during feeding. Only one person is needed for feeding. The child is unable to sit with a hip spica cast in place.

Client Need: Health Promotion and Maintenance

7.   The nurse is to administer Lasix 40 mg intramuscularly. The vial reads 100 mg in 5 ml. How many milliliters should the nurse administer?

_____

Answer: 2

Rationale: A ratio and proportion formula is used to show that 100 mg is to 5 ml as 40 mg is to X milliliters. The answer is 2 milliliters.

Client Need: Physiological Integrity

> **Did you remember *not* to label your answer? The question asked how many milliliters the nurse should administer.**

8.   An adolescent was involved in an after-school fight and comes to the emergency room complaining of multiple bruises and a bite to his right forearm. The skin is broken and the bleeding is controlled. His last tetanus shot was 8 ½ years ago. The nurse's priority action is to do which of the following?

1. Assess for signs of internal bleeding.
2. Administer 0.5 ml of tetanus toxoid intramuscularly.
3. Notify the authorities of the assault.
4. Prepared to suture the skin closed.

Answer: 2

Rationale: A tetanus shot is indicated because there has not been a timely booster. There is no indication of internal bleeding. There is no need to contact the police. The bleeding is controlled, and suturing is not necessary.

Client Need: Physiological Integrity

---

9. The mother of a terminally ill child tells the nurse she wants to take her child home. Which of the following is the nurse's **best** response?

1. "Tell me why you want to take your child home."
2. "The pediatrician is the only one who can discharge your child."
3. "You have not given the medication a chance to work."
4. "I will help you get ready to leave."

Answer: 1

Rationale: In an upsetting situation such as this, it is best for the nurse to try and get the mother to express her needs and concerns. She cannot be stopped from signing her child out against medical advice, and the nurse has an obligation to explain the ramifications of the mother's actions to her.

Client Need: Psychosocial Integrity

---

10. A client in the first stage of labor is being monitored by the labor and delivery room nurse. The client has an external fetal monitor and has intravenous fluids infusing. After 3 hours of labor the nurse notes variable decelerations in the fetal heart rate on the monitoring strip. The nurse knows that variable deceleration's are caused by compression of the

_____.

Answer: Umbilical cord

Rationale: Variable decelerations are caused by compression of the fetal umbilical cord. **Ea**rly decelerations are caused by fetal h**ea**d compression. **La**te decelerations are caused by uterop**la**cental insufficiency.

> Did you remember that variable decelerations are caused by fetal *umbilical* cord compression?

Client Need: Physiological Integrity

---

11. A classic integumentary sign and symptom of hyperbilirubinemia in the newborn infant is known as _____.

Answer: Physiological jaundice

Rationale: Jaundice in the newborn usually manifests in the first 2 to 4 days of life. It is treated with hydration and phototherapy.

Client Need: Physiological Integrity

---

12. A client with emphysema is at home and is having difficulty with mobility. He spends most of his day in a reclining chair. Which physiological response to prolonged immobility would a nurse expect to assess?

1. Increased insulin production.
2. Decreased red blood cell production.
3. Decreased sodium excretion.
4. Increased calcium excretion.

Answer: 4

Rationale: Prolonged immobility leads to the breakdown of bone tissue. This results in increased calcium excretion. Immobility does not increase insulin production, decrease red blood cell production, or decrease sodium excretion.

Client Need: Physiological Integrity

13.   A 6-month-old is admitted to the hospital with dehydration. The infant's admission weight is 15 pounds. Which of the following parameters indicates to the nurse that the infant has a normal urinary output?

1.   1 to 2 ml urine output per kilogram of body weight per hour.
2.   10 to 12 ml urine output per kilogram of body weight per hour.
3.   7.5 ml urine output per kilogram of body weight per hour.
4.   15 ml urine output per kilogram of body weight per hour.

Answer: 1

Rationale: The normal urinary output for infants is 1 to 2 ml urine output per kilogram of body weight per hour. The other answers are wrong and would indicate excessive fluid loss.

Client Need: Physiological Integrity

14.   A nursing instructor is teaching a class of students about neurological assessment of newborns. Which of the following findings indicate to the nurse that the newborn is neurologically healthy? Select all that apply.

1.   The neonate turns to the nurse when the cheek is brushed.
2.   The newborn does not respond to loud noises.
3.   The neonate has a poor suck reflex.
4.   The newborn grasps the nurse's finger when the palm of the hand is touched.
5.   The newborn steps when held over a flat surface with soles of feet touching.

Answers: 1, 4, and 5

Rationale: A newborn who turns to the nurse when the cheek is brushed is displaying the rooting reflex. Grasping the nurse's finger when the palm of the hand is touched and stepping when held over a flat surface are normal neurological signs. A newborn who does not respond to loud noises and has a poor suck reflex needs further neurological assessment.

Client Need: Health Promotion and Maintenance

15. A 50-year-old client is admitted with a diagnosis of acute osteomyelitis of the right leg. She is complaining of acute pain, especially when she ambulates. Her temperature is 101.8°F, and there is a red warm area on her right calf. Based on the nurse's assessment, which of the following nursing diagnoses is most appropriate for this client?

1. High risk for infection related to right leg irritation.
2. Altered nutrition, less than body requirements related to the need for the client to remain NPO.
3. Activity intolerance related to acute severe leg pain.
4. Sensory deprivation related to need to keep client in isolation.

Answer: 3

Rationale: The assessment reveals that the client has severe pain when walking. The other diagnoses are not supported in the assessment.

Client Needs: Physiological Integrity

> Did you remember that the first sign and symptom discussed in the question was a priority sign and symptom to be addressed in the answer?

16. A woman who is 15 weeks pregnant comes to the obstetrics clinic to have an amniocentesis. The nurse knows this test is used to identify which of the following traits or problems? Select all that apply.

1. Surfactant level.
2. Cephalopelvic disproportion.
3. Genetic defects.
4. Neural tube defects.
5. Sex of the fetus.

Answers: 3, 4, and 5

Rationale: Amniotic fluid may be tested for chromosome defects, neural tube defects, and the sex of the fetus. Surfactant levels are tested in the second and third trimesters. Cephalopelvic disproportion is diagnosed by x-ray or abdominal ultrasound in the third trimester.

Client Need: Physiological Integrity

17. A postoperative client is returned to your unit. You as the nurse know that which of the following nursing interventions is the most important in preventing pneumonia for your client?

1. Administer oxygen via nasal cannula as ordered by the physician.
2. Have the client cough, deep breathe, and change position every 4 hours.
3. Administer pain medications before coughing and deep breathing exercises, and encourage the client to use the incentive spirometer.
4. Administer intravenous antibiotics every 4 hours as ordered by the surgeon.

Answer: 3

Rationale: Preventing pneumonia is easiest when the client coughs and deep breathes regularly and uses the incentive spirometer as ordered. Clients are better able to complete these tasks when pain is minimized.

> This answer is the most comprehensive. Also, step 5 works here.

Client Need: Physiological Integrity

18. A 5-year-old child is admitted to the pediatric unit with a diagnosis of acute rheumatic fever. The nurse asks the mother which of the following appropriate questions?

1. "Has your child had a sore throat recently?"
2. "Was your child born with this cardiac defect?"
3. "Do you know who gave your child this infection?"
4. "Are you aware that your child will be placed on isolation precautions for the next 10 days?"

Answer: 1

Rationale: Rheumatic fever is associated with streptococcal infections, such as a strep throat. It is not a cardiac defect nor does the child get it from others. There is no reason for the child to be in isolation.

Client Need: Physiological Integrity

19. The nurse is to administer Kefzol 100 mg intravenously in 100 ml of D5 water over a 20-minute period. The drop factor on the tubing is 15. At what rate would the nurse set the infusion pump?

_____

Answer: 75 gtts per minute

Rationale: The flow rate is determined by the amount of solution (100 ml) divided by the infusion time in minutes (20) and then multiplied by the drop factor (15).

Client Need: Physiological Integrity

> Did you remember to label your answer in drops per minute? The question asked what the flow rate was and did not specify the label.

20. A pregnant client is at risk for developing preeclampsia. The nurse knows the _priority_ assessment for this client includes which of the following? Select all that apply.

1. Glycosuria.
2. Proteinuria.
3. Edema.
4. Hypertension.
5. Hyperreflexia.
6. Bradycardia.

Answers: 2, 3, and 4

Rationale: The three cardinal signs and symptoms of preeclampsia are proteinuria, hypertension, and edema with weight gain. Glycosuria is associated with gestational diabetes.

Client Need: Health Promotion and Maintenance

21. A postoperative client with a nasogastric tube has had 2500 ml of drainage since the beginning of the nurse's shift. The nurse must be especially alert for which of the following electrolyte imbalances?

1. Elevated sodium level.
2. Decreased potassium level.
3. Elevated magnesium level.
4. Decreased calcium level.

Answer: 2

Rationale: Loss of fluid from the stomach is a common cause of potassium depletion. The other electrolyte imbalances are not associated with intestinal fluid loss.

Client Need: Physiological Integrity

22. A child with sickle cell anemia is being discharged after an acute crisis episode. Which of the following should the nurse include as part of the teaching plan for the child's parents?

1. Monitor the child's temperature daily.
2. Restrict outdoor play activity to 1 hour per day.
3. Encourage the child to drink lots of fluids.
4. Have the child eat a high-protein diet.

Answer: 3

Rationale: Preventing dehydration is an important step in preventing a sickle cell crisis. The child's temperature should be monitored only when fever is suspected. The child can play as usual and eat a healthy balanced diet.

> Did you try using step 5 with this question?

Client Need: Physiological Integrity

---

23. Clients who experience hypokalemia related to nausea, vomiting, and diarrhea exhibit which of the following signs and symptoms?

1. Confusion.
2. Thirst.
3. Arrhythmia.
4. Muscles spasms.

Answer: 3

Rationale: An irregular pulse is a clinical manifestation of hypokalemia. Confusion is associated with hyponatremia. Thirst is associated with hypernatremia

> If you did not know the answer to this question, you could have chosen the answer that is most *life threatening* or used step 5.

Client Need: Physiological Integrity

---

24. A newly delivered first time mother asks the nurse how to tell if her baby hears well. She explains that the baby's maternal grandmother was born deaf. Which response by the nurse is best?

1. "There is no need to worry. Deafness is not inherited."
2. "Your pediatrician will test your baby's hearing."
3. "Most states now mandate screening tests for hearing on newborns. Your baby has passed."
4. "The best way to determine if your baby can hear is to clap your hands loudly and see if the baby startles."

Answer: 3

Rationale: Mandatory hearing screening is done in most states. It is inappropriate for the nurse to tell the mother not to worry and to assure the mother that her infant can hear. Clapping hands is an unreliable way of testing hearing.

Client Need: Health Promotion and Maintenance

25.   A postoperative client returns to the unit in skeletal traction. The nurse expects to assess which of the following? Select all that apply.

1. Slight pain at the insertion site.
2. Serous drainage on the dressing.
3. Movement of the pin at the insertion site.
4. Ace bandages securely wrapped around the traction ropes.
5. Minimal edema around the pin.

Answers: 1, 2, and 5

Rationale: Skeletal pins that move should be reported to the surgeon immediately. It is normal to expect minor pain and minimal edema. In the early postoperative period serous drainage is also anticipated. Ace bandages wrapped over the ropes do not allow the traction apparatus to work correctly.

Client Need: Physiological Integrity

26. Children who grind their teeth, especially during sleep, are said to have what disorder?

_____

Answer: Bruxism

Rationale: Bruxism can be so severe that the child's teeth may be damaged and worn down.

Client Need: Physiological Integrity

27. A 60-year-old woman is to have a left lobectomy for lung cancer. She tells the nurse that she is scared and wishes she had never smoked. What is the nurse's *most* appropriate response?

1. "It's okay to feel afraid. Let's talk about what you are afraid of."
2. "Don't worry. The important thing is you have now quit smoking."
3. "I understand your fears. I was a smoker also."
4. "Your doctor is a great surgeon. You will be fine."

Answer: 1

Rationale: It is the nurse's responsibility to acknowledge the client's statement and encourage verbalization. It is not the nurse's responsibility to tell the client not to worry or to tell a client he or she understands the client's feelings. It is inappropriate to tell a client he or she will be fine.

Client Need: Psychosocial Integrity

28. A client with an internal repair of a right hip fracture is being discharged home. The nurse knows that teaching has been effective when the client tells the nurse that he will rest during the day sitting on what piece of furniture?

1. A reclining chair with an ottoman.
2. A straight-backed chair with an elevated seat.
3. A couch with plush cushions.
4. A rocking chair with a curved back.

Answer: 2

Rationale: A straight-backed chair with an elevated seat allows the client to assume proper positioning when sitting. An elevated seat decreases the risk of his hip dislocation. The other options do not support a proper posture and may cause hip dislocation.

Client Need: Physiological Integrity

29. The nurse is making a home visit for an adolescent who attempted suicide. The parents tell the nurse their son is doing well. Which of the following behaviors, if reported by the parents, would cause the nurse to be alarmed? The adolescent is

1. Talking on his cell phone with friends.
2. Anxious to return to school.
3. Eating meals normally.
4. Planning to give his CD collection to his girlfriend.

Answer: 4

Rationale: Giving away favorite possessions has always been associated with ideas of suicide and suicide plans. The other answers demonstrate a return to normal adolescent behavior.

Client Need: Psychosocial Integrity

30. Which of the following responses by the nurse is the most appropriate for the newly delivered mother whose newborn has died in the delivery room?

1. "I understand your grief. I lost a baby also."
2. "You may hold your baby as long as you want."
3. "I have called for the chaplain to come and stay with you."
4. "This is for the best. Your baby was very ill."

Answer: 2

Rationale: When a newborn dies, the mother is encouraged to stay with the baby as long as she wants. A photo can also be taken of the baby. The nurse should not personalize answers nor leave the mother alone.

Client Need: Psychosocial Integrity

31. The nurse is to administer ampicillin 500 mg intramuscularly. After reconstituting the ampicillin, the solution available is 1 g per 5 ml. How many milliliters should the nurse administer?

Answer: 2.5

Rationale: 1 g is equivalent to 1000 mg. The nurse needs half that amount. The formula used is 500 mg divided by 1000 mg multiplied by 5 ml.

> **Did you remember *not* to label your answer? The label was part of the stem of the question.**

Client Need: Physiological Integrity

32. The client in the first trimester of pregnancy comes to the clinic to be evaluated. The client states, "I am so nauseous, I vomit all day long." The nurse knows that the client should be evaluated for which complication associated with the first trimester of pregnancy?

Answer: Hyperemesis gravidarum

Rationale: Women in the first trimester of pregnancy who excessively vomit are at risk for dehydration and starvation. These women must be treated and watched for signs of fluid and electrolyte imbalances and malnutrition.

Client Need: Physiological Integrity

33.   The parents of a child with a suppressed immune system ask the nurse how to determine if the child has an infection. The nurse tells the parents to look for which of the following signs and symptoms?

1. Loss of appetite.
2. Restlessness and irritability.
3. Complaints of a stomach ache.
4. Elevated temperature greater than 100.5°F.

Answer: 4

Rationale: A fever is a cardinal sign and symptom of infection. The other answers are not typically associated with infection.

Client Need: Physiological Integrity

34.   The nurse assesses a client and determines that the client is in the **compensatory** stage of shock. Which behavior has the nurse **most** likely observed?

1. Confusion.
2. Garbled speech.
3. Unconsciousness.
4. Restlessness.

Answer: 4

Rationale: Restlessness is seen in the compensatory stage of shock. Confusion is seen in the progressive stage of shock, and garbled speech and unconsciousness are seen in the irreversible stage of shock.

Did you remember that compensatory is an early stage of shock?

Client Need: Physiological Integrity

35. Which of the following is the best indicator that peristalsis is returning to normal for the postoperative appendectomy client?

1. Hypoactive bowel sounds are auscultated in two quadrants.
2. The client asks for a cup of tea and some toast.
3. The client passes flatus.
4. Abdominal palpation does not reveal rigidity.

Answer: 3

Rationale: Passing flatus and belching indicate the return of peristaltic activity. Hyperactive bowel sounds should be heard. Hunger and thirst do not indicate the return of peristaltic activity, nor does lack of rigidity.

Client Need: Physiological Integrity

36. A primiparous mother newly delivered is breastfeeding her newborn. She asks the nurse when her breastmilk will come in. The nurse most appropriately responds with which of the following?

1. In 1 to 2 days.
2. In 2 to 4 days.
3. In 4 to 5 days.
4. In 5 to 6 days.

Answer: 2

Rationale: Colostrum is used to nourish newborns for the first 36 to 48 hours. In 48 to 96 hours the mother's milk supply is established.

Client Need: Health Promotion and Maintenance

37. A malabsorption syndrome of the intestinal tract characterized by diarrhea, malnutrition, bleeding tendencies, and hypocalcemia is known as

_____.

Answer: Celiac disease

Rationale: Clients with this disease are taught to eat diets free of gluten. Gluten is a protein found in whole wheat and other grains.

Client Need: Physiological Integrity

38.   A client taking lithium is to be discharged home. The nurse teaches the client which of the following important dietary considerations for lithium therapy?

   1. Eat a diet high in sodium.
   2. Eat a diet low in potassium.
   3. Maintain adequate sodium in the diet.
   4. Increase potassium in the diet.

Answer: 3

Rationale: Lithium is a salt. If the client's sodium level falls, lithium will be retained and the client will be at risk for lithium toxicity.

Client Need: Physiological Integrity

Were you able to apply step 4 to this question? Answers 1, 2, and 4 instruct the client to raise or lower electrolyte intake while answer 3 has the client maintain sodium intake.

39.   A 28-year-old client is admitted in active labor at 39 weeks gestation. The nurse assesses the fetus and locates the heart rate above the umbilicus, midline. The nurse correctly suspects the fetus is in which of the following positions?

   1. Cephalic.
   2. Transverse.
   3. Posterior.
   4. Frank breech.

Answer: 4

Rationale: With Frank breech presentation, the fetal heart rate is above the level of the umbilicus. In cephalic, transverse, and posterior presentations the fetal heart rate is located in areas below the umbilicus.

Client Need: Health Promotion and Maintenance

40.   A client is suspected of having cancer of the lungs. He is admitted for a bronchoscopy with biopsy. After the procedure the nurse completes which of the following as priority interventions?

1. Monitor the client's breathing and assess for signs of pneumothorax.
2. Keep client NPO and allow the client to gargle with oral lidocaine to decrease pain.
3. Administer intravenous solutions and oxygen as ordered by the physician.
4. Provide the client with a pad and pencil and discourage talking for 4 hours.

Answer: 1

Rationale: A client having a bronchoscopy with biopsy is at risk for pneumothorax. Gargling with lidocaine will not allow the gag reflex to return. Intravenous solutions and oxygen administration will not prevent a pneumothorax. The client can speak after the procedure.

> Did you remember Airway, Breathing, Circulation?

Client Need: Physiological Integrity

41.   A client in the cardiac care unit is to receive intravenous fluids at 100 ml per hour. The drop factor on the tubing is 60. At what rate should the nurse set the infusion pump?

_____

Answer: 100 drops per minute

Rationale: When using microtubing, the milliliters per hour equal the drops per minute. The formula is volume (100 ml) divided by the time (60 minutes) multiplied by the drop factor (60).

Client Need: Physiological Integrity

> Did you remember to label your answer? The question did not ask for drops per minute. This information is something you must supply in your answer.

---

42. The nurse is teaching a class of young women about birth control methods. When discussing birth control pills, it is important for the nurse to point out that certain medications decrease the efficiency of the pill. These medications include which of the following?

1. Analgesics.
2. Diuretics.
3. Antibiotics.
4. Antihistamines.

Answer: 3

Rationale: Client's taking broad-spectrum antibiotics and birth control pills should include additional birth control methods to avoid unwanted pregnancies.

Client Need: Physiological Integrity

> Did you use "true" and "false" or step 5 for this *fact* question?

---

43. The nurse is to administer digoxin 0.25 mg by mouth every morning. The digoxin comes in scored tablets of 0.125 mg each. What is the correct dosage for the nurse to administer?

> Did you remember to label your answer? The question did not provide you with a dosing label.

_____

Answer: 2 tablets

Rationale: When you add 0.125 mg plus 0.125 mg, you get 0.25 mg. Hence, the nurse must give 2 tablets.

Client Need: Safe Effective Care Environment

> **Did you see the unnecessary information provided in the question? Stating that the tablets were scored was information you did not need.**

---

44. A nurse enters a client's room and finds the client pulseless. The family has requested a do not resuscitate order from the physician but the order has not been written to date. What is the nurse's **most** appropriate action?

1. Call a code.
2. Begin cardiopulmonary resuscitation without calling a code.
3. Call the physician stat for a do not resuscitate order.
4. Respect the family's wishes and do nothing.

Answer: 1

Rationale: Unless the physician writes a do not resuscitate order, the nurse is obligated to call a code.

Client Need: Physiological Integrity

---

45. A client who is 36 weeks pregnant is being monitored in the antepartum unit. She has been diagnosed with pregnancy-induced hypertension. Suddenly, the client complains of continuous abdominal pain and vaginal bleeding. The nurse knows the client is probably experiencing which of the following complications?

1. Placenta previa.
2. Prolapsed cord.
3. Ruptured ovarian cysts.
4. Abruptio placentae.

Answer: 4

Rationale: The cardinal signs and symptoms of abruptio placentae include a rigid board-like abdomen, severe pain, and heavy vaginal bleeding. Placenta previa occurs with painless vaginal bleeding.

Client Need: Physiological Integrity

46.   A 58-year-old woman is returned from the postanesthesia care unit after a subtotal thyroidectomy. The client's vital signs are stable and her dressing is dry. The nurse correctly positions the client in which of the following positions?

   1.   High Fowler's with her neck flexed.
   2.   High Fowler's with her neck erect.
   3.   Semi-Fowler's with her neck flexed.
   4.   Semi-Fowler's with her neck erect.

Answer: 4

Rationale: Placing the client in a semi-Fowler's position with the neck erect assists in maintaining a patent airway. Flexing the neck may compromise the airway.

Client Need: Physiological Integrity

> **Did you remember that semi-Fowler's is the position of choice for most postoperative clients? Also, an erect neck opens the airway.**

47.   A 78-year-old woman fell in her home and is admitted to your unit with a fractured femoral head. Skin traction is ordered to help reduce the fracture. Twenty-four hours after admission, the client begins to experience shortness of breath and dyspnea. The nurse correctly determines the client has developed which of the following complications?

   1.   Pneumonia.
   2.   Pulmonary fat embolism.
   3.   Pneumothorax.
   4.   Mediastinal shift.

Answer: 2

Rationale: Pulmonary fat embolism is associated with fractures of long bones. Pneumonia is associated with immobility.

Client Need: Physiological Integrity

48.   A client admitted for abdominal surgery states that he is very anxious about the operation. A **priority** nursing intervention for this client is to do which of the following?

    1.   Ask him to describe what he is feeling.
    2.   Reassure him he will be fine.
    3.   Suggest he concentrate on other thoughts.
    4.   Refer him to the pastoral care team.

Answer: 1

Rationale: The nurse is responsible for assisting clients to express themselves and explore feelings. You cannot offer reassurance. Answers 3 and 4 are not applicable.

Client Need: Psychosocial Integrity

49.   The mother of a 2-year-old calls the pediatric clinic to report that her child has a viral infection and is febrile. She asks the nurse how many baby aspirin she should give to the toddler. The nurse's **best** response is to tell the mother to do which of the following?

    1.   Give the child three baby aspirin every 4 hours as needed.
    2.   Follow the directions on the label according to the child's weight.
    3.   Give the child Tylenol and not aspirin.
    4.   Bring the child to the clinic to be assessed.

Answer: 3

Rationale: From infancy to the age of adolescence, children should take Tylenol and not aspirin due to its relationship with Reye's syndrome.

Client Need: Physiological Integrity

50. A nursing instructor is preparing a group of students to care for clients on the psychiatric ward. The instructor assigns a student to a client who is admitted because he has broken off normal thought processes from his consciousness. This disorder is known as _____.

Answer: Dissociation

Rationale: Dissociation is seen in clients with amnesia, conversion reaction, or as a result of taking certain medications.

Client Need: Psychosocial Integrity

51. The nurse caring for a client on contact isolation is exiting the room. Number in sequence the order in which the nurse would complete the following tasks to leave the room according to protocol.

___ Wash hands.
___ Remove gloves.
___ Untie gown at waist.
___ Remove gown.
___ Untie gown at back of neck.

Answer: 5, 2, 1, 4, 3

Rationale: The nurse would first untie the isolation gown at the waist and then remove gloves. Next, untie the gown at the back of the neck and then remove the gown. Washing hands is done last as the nurse leaves the room.

Client Need: Health Promotion and Maintenance

52.   The nurse is teaching a client newly diagnosed with type 1 diabetes about controlling blood sugar levels. The nurse knows the teaching has been successful when the client states which of the following?

1. "I will control my blood sugar level by eating healthy."
2. "I will keep my blood sugar level down by exercising every day."
3. "I will take my diabetic pills every morning to maintain a low blood glucose level."
4. "I will take my insulin injections as ordered to help control blood glucose levels."

Answer: 4

Rationale: A type 1 diabetic must take insulin injections every day. Oral medications work for type 2 diabetics. Exercise and diet are important but not the priority.

Client Need: Health Promotion and Maintenance

53.   A 32-year-old man is admitted to the hospital with a diagnosis of renal calculi. The nurse receives the physician's orders and determines which of the following is the **priority** intervention?

1. Strain all urine.
2. Schedule an intravenous pyelogram.
3. Keep on strict intake and output.
4. Send client for an abdominal ultrasound.

Answer: 1

Rationale: The priority nursing action for a client with renal calculi is to strain all urine to determine if there is passage of a renal stone. The other admission orders are important but not the priority.

Client Need: Physiological Integrity

54.   The nurse knows clients receiving steroid therapy should be given their daily dose of the medication at which of the following times?

1. At night with water.
2. In the morning with milk.
3. In the afternoon on an empty stomach.
4. In the evening before dinner.

Answer: 2

Rationale: Steroids can be taken in the morning with milk to decrease the chance of gastrointestinal upset. Steroids should never be taken on an empty stomach.

Client Need: Physiological Integrity

55.   The nurse is assessing the client for signs and symptoms of hypoxia. A good indication of this condition is which of the following?

1. Bradycardia.
2. Hypertension.
3. Hyperthermia.
4. Cyanosis.

Answer: 4

Rationale: Cyanosis, especially of the mucosal lining, is a good indication of hypoxia. Many clients also suffer with tachycardia and hypotension. Body temperature is not necessarily affected.

Client Need: Physiological Integrity

56.   A 50-year-old woman comes to the women's health clinic. She tells the nurse she has had an irregular menses for the past year and occasional hot flashes and mood swings. She wants to know when she can stop using birth control. The nurse's best response is which of the following?

1. "You must continue using birth control until you have missed 24 consecutive menses cycles."
2. "You may stop now because it has been a year since you were regular with your menses."
3. "You must wait 6 more months before you can stop using birth control."
4. "You should continue using birth control until the age of 55 to be safe."

Answer: 1

Rationale: A woman who misses 24 consecutive menstrual cycles does not need to continue using birth control. Irregular cycles are not considered criteria for stopping birth control. The age for women to stop using birth control varies.

Client Need: Health Promotion and Maintenance

57. An adolescent hospitalized with anorexia nervosa is scheduled for discharge. The nurse knows that a good indication that the client has improved is which of the following?

1. She no longer purges after a meal.
2. She requests to start an exercise regimen.
3. She has gained 4 pounds.
4. She talks about returning to school.

Answer: 3

Rationale: A weight gain of 4 pounds is a good indication that the client is eating. Clients with bulimia purge after meals. Exercise and wanting to return to school are not indicators of improvement.

Did you use step 5 for this question?

Client Need: Psychosocial Integrity

58. An antepartum client at 36 weeks gestation is admitted to the labor and delivery unit for observation. She has been diagnosed with pregnancy-induced hypertension. Within 4 hours of admission she suffers a seizure and lapses into a coma. The nurse anticipates the client will be diagnosed with what disorder?

     _____

     Answer: Eclampsia

     Rationale: Eclampsia usually develops when a woman with preeclampsia is not treated or is treated unsuccessfully. It is often characterized by a seizure and/or coma. This condition can be fatal if untreated.

     Client Need: Physiological Integrity

59. Clients with airborne diseases are usually placed on respiratory precautions. The nurse is aware that the protective equipment **most** important to use is which of the following?

     1. A mask.
     2. Gloves.
     3. Gown.
     4. Goggles.

     Answer: 1

     Rationale: The most important piece of protective equipment a nurse must use when caring for a client on respiratory precautions is a mask.

     Ah-ha question! Did you remember to stretch and take some deep breaths?

     Client Need: Safe Effective Care Environment

60. The 28-year-old man who was hit in the head has just returned from the operating room for evacuation of a subdural hematoma. The **priority** nursing intervention is which of the following?

1. Observe for signs of increased intracranial pressure.
2. Assess for leakage of cerebral spinal fluid.
3. Assess for intracranial hemorrhaging.
4. Maintain a patent airway.

Answer: 4

Rationale: Maintenance of a patent airway is the priority answer. The other answers are all important to perform but are not the priority.

Client Need: Physiological Integrity

> Here is an example of a question that has four correct answers. If you remembered that the ABCs, airway, breathing, and circulation, are your priority, you got it right.

61. The mother of a 5-year-old child with cystic fibrosis is learning about the purpose of pancreatic enzymes. The nurse understands that further teaching is necessary when the mother states which of the following?

1. "I will give my son the enzymes after each meal."
2. "I will give my son the enzymes before each meal."
3. "The enzymes are helpful in the digestion of fat."
4. "I will put the enzyme crystals in applesauce to give to my son."

Answer: 1

Rationale: Pancreatic enzymes are given before each meal. The enzymes aid in the digestion of fat and can be given with nonfat foods such as applesauce.

Client Need: Physiological Integrity

62. An emergency room nurse admits a client with a deep gash of the left forearm. What priority nursing intervention should the nurse complete?

1. Apply a tourniquet below the left elbow and release every 5 minutes.
2. Elevate the arm and apply ice to the wound.
3. Clean the wound and prepare for suturing.
4. Apply direct pressure over the wound.

Answer: 4

Rationale: The priority nursing intervention is to apply direct pressure to the wound to stop the bleeding. After controlling bleeding, the wound can be cleansed and prepared for suturing. A tourniquet is not appropriate at this time.

Client Need: Physiological Integrity

63. A term client in labor comes to the labor and delivery unit and states that she has saturated two perineal pads in the past 30 minutes. The nurse suspects placenta previa. The priority nursing action is to complete which of the following?

1. Examine the client to determine effacement and dilatation.
2. Place the client on external fetal monitoring.
3. Prepare the client to begin pushing.
4. Notify the obstetrician.

Answer: 4

Rationale: There are no vaginal exams done on clients with suspected or known placenta previa. The obstetrician needs to be called because an emergency cesarean section is probable.

Client Need: Physiological Integrity

64.   A nurse is bathing a 1-year-old child and notices a large abdominal mass. It is also noted that the child's diaper has pink-tinged urine. The nurse correctly suspects the child has which of the following diagnoses?

   1. Pyloric stenosis.
   2. Nephrosis.
   3. Wilms' tumor.
   4. Intussusception.

   Answer: 3

   Rationale: Wilms' tumors are most often characterized by an abdominal mass and hematuria. Pyloric stenosis and intussusception are disorders of the gastrointestinal tract. Nephrosis does not cause an abdominal mass.

   Client Need: Physiological Integrity

65.   A 42-year-old man is admitted to the nursing unit from the emergency room with a diagnosis of detached retina OS (left eye). Which of the following physician orders should the nurse anticipate?

   1. Keep both eyes patched.
   2. Place the client in a low Fowler's position.
   3. Turn the client to a left lateral position.
   4. Instill eye drops every 4 hours as ordered.

   Answer: 1

   Rationale: It is important to minimize eye movement preoperatively. Patching both eyes helps to accomplish this. The head of the bed should be in a semi- to high Fowler's position. The client should not be turned to the side and will not receive eye drops until after surgery.

   Client Need: Physiological Integrity

66.   A client is to receive codeine ¼ grain by mouth stat. The nurse would correctly administer how many milligrams?

_____

Answer: 15

Rationale: 1 grain is equivalent to 60 mg. Therefore ¼ grain is equivalent to 15 mg.

Client Need: Safe Effective Care Environment

67.   A 2-month-old infant has undergone repair of a cleft palate. The nurse knows the **priority** nursing intervention in the immediate postoperative period is which of the following?

1. Feeding the infant half-strength formula for the first 48 hours.
2. Applying and releasing elbow restraints every 2 hours.
3. Preventing inflammation of the suture line.
4. Suctioning the nasopharynx frequently.

Did you remember client safety for this question?

Answer: 2

Rationale: The infant will start full-strength formula within 12 hours of surgery. Elbow restraints must be used to prevent disruption to the suture line. Inflammation of the suture line will occur later on postoperatively. Suctioning is not done frequently.

Client Need: Physiological Integrity

68.   A multiparous woman delivered a healthy baby girl 8 hours ago. During assessment the nurse assists the client to the bathroom to void. Which of the following symptoms alerted the nurse to the client's need to void?

1. Moderate lochia rubra.
2. Fundus three finger breaths above the umbilicus.
3. Swelling of the labia.
4. Maternal heart rate of 61.

Answer: 2

Rationale: A full bladder will most often raise the level of uterine fundus and possibly deviate it to the side. The other answers are not associated with a full bladder.

Client Need: Health Promotion and Maintenance

69.   A postoperative client has an intravenous order as follows:

Bag 1: 1000 ml Ringer's lactate.
Bag 2: 1000 ml D$_5$W normal saline.
Bag 3: 1000 ml D$_5$W.

The solutions are to infuse in 24 hours. Drop factor of the tubing is 10. The nurse correctly sets the infusion pump to run at how many drops per minute?

_____

Answer: 21

Rationale: 3000 ml in 24 hours equates to 125 ml an hour (3000 divided by 24). This number divided by 60 minutes multiplied by the drop factor of 10 gives you the correct answer of 21 drops per minute.

Did you remember *not* to label your answer because the label was included in the question?

Client Need: Safe Effective Care Environment

70.   A 54-year-old woman with Ménière's disease is admitted to the hospital because of increasingly more frequent and serious episodes of vertigo. She asks the nurse if she can use the bathroom whenever she wants. The nurse appropriately responds with which of the following comments?

1. "No. You are on strict bed rest."
2. "Yes, you can use the bathroom whenever you want to."
3. "You will have to speak to your physician about that."
4. "You will need to ring your bell for assistance whenever you get out of bed."

Answer: 4

Rationale: The client must have someone with her to avoid a fall. Safety is paramount for the client.

Client Need: Safe Effective Care Environment

---

71.   A client is to receive 250 mg of an antibiotic intramuscularly. The vial reads 3 g in 5 ml. The nurse correctly draws how many milliliters for injection?

_____

Answer: 0.4

Rationale: A ratio proportion formula is used. 3000 mg, which is equal to 3 g, is to 5 ml as 250 mg is to X milliliters. The correct answer is 0.4 ml.

> **Did you remember *not to* label your answer because the label was included in the question?**

Client Need: Health Promotion and Maintenance

---

72.   A 65-year-old man is admitted to the cardiac care unit. A diagnosis of myocardial infarction is made, and the client is placed on a cardiac monitor. An intravenous solution of D_5RL is infusing at 50 ml per hour. The client's vital signs are stable, and he is requesting to see his wife. The nurse's **priority** assessment for this client is which of the following?

1. Apical pulse rate.
2. Respiratory rate.
3. Blood pressure.
4. Chest pain.

Answer: 4

Rationale: The priority concern for a client with myocardial infarction is to assess the presence of chest pain. The

> **Are you paying attention to words that are in bold, *italics*, or are underlined? Remember, they should be used to help you find the correct answer.**

client's vital signs are stable so it is not necessary to reassess answers 1, 2, and 3.

Client Need: Physiological Integrity

. . . .

73.   A postpartum client who delivered 7 days ago calls the clinic complaining of pain and redness of the left calf. The nurse advises the client to do which of the following? Select all that apply.

1. Call her physician.
2. Massage the area.
3. Elevate her leg.
4. Apply warmth to the affected area.
5. Decrease leg movement as much as possible.

Answers: 1, 3, 4, and 5

Rationale: Elevation, warmth, and decreasing movement are all appropriate with a suspected diagnosis of deep vein thrombosis. Notifying the physician is also appropriate. Massage is not done as it could dislocate the clot.

Client Need: Physiological Integrity

. . . .

74.   A cardiac client is to receive lidocaine intravenously. The nurse adds 2 g of lidocaine to 500 ml of D5W. To infuse at 2 mg per minute, the nurse would set the infusion pump at how many milliliters per hour?

_____

Answer: 30

Rationale: There are 2 mg of lidocaine in 0.5 ml of solution. A ratio and proportion formula shows that 2000 mg (2 g) is to 500 ml as 2 mg is to *X* milliliters. If the client is to have 2 mg per minute or 0.5 ml per minute, you multiply this by 60 (minutes), which equals 120 mg per hour or 30 ml per hour.

Client Need: Physiological Integrity

. . . .

75.   The nurse is instructing a class of nursing students on how to determine the estimated date of delivery for a pregnant woman. Which of the following are acceptable methods to use in determining the estimated date of delivery? Select all that apply.

1. A nonstress test.
2. Naegele's rule.
3. Ultrasonography.
4. Oxytocin challenge test.
5. Audible fetal heart tones.

Answers: 2, 3, and 5

Rationale: Naegele's rule, ultrasound, and fetal heart tones are all acceptable methods for determining estimated date of delivery. A nonstress test and oxytocin challenge tests are done for other reasons late in pregnancy.

Client Need: Health Promotion and Maintenance

76.   A 30-year-old woman is brought to the psychiatric emergency room with complaints of feeling depressed, moody, and overly anxious. She tells the nurse she has experienced feelings of sadness and gloom recently. She is asking for help. As part of the admission process, what is the nurse's **priority** assessment?

1. The client's home environment.
2. The client's support systems.
3. The client's suicide risk.
4. The client's past psychiatric history.

Answer: 3

Rationale: The priority assessment is the client's thoughts and/or plans for suicide. Keeping the client safe is the main concern. It is also important to assess the home environment, her support systems, and past psychiatric history, but these are not the priority at this time.

Client Need: Psychosocial Integrity

77. A breastfeeding mother asks the nurse about what changes she should make in her diet to ensure an adequate supply of healthy breast milk. The nurse suggests which of the following?

1. Increasing her caloric intake by 1000 calories a day.
2. Decreasing her fat intake.
3. Consuming four to five glasses of milk a day.
4. Avoiding red meats and shellfish.

Answer: 3

Rationale: The lactating mother should consume four to five servings of milk a day or the equivalent. The increase in calories necessary is 200 to 300 a day. There is no need to decrease fat consumption or to avoid red meat and shellfish.

Client Need: Health Promotion and Maintenance

78. A 36-year-old man is admitted with a diagnosis of cirrhosis of the liver secondary to alcoholism. He is underweight and has ascites and portal hypertension. The physician orders neomycin. The nurse understands the desired effect of this drug is to do which of the following?

1. Decrease serum ammonia levels.
2. Boost the client's immune system.
3. Reverse the ascites.
4. Neutralize intestinal flora.

Answer: 1

Rationale: The purpose of neomycin is to decrease the client's serum ammonia levels. Answers 2, 3, and 4 are not associated with use of neomycin.

Client Need: Physiological Integrity

79.   The parents of a 16-year-old, brought to the emergency room after taking a bottle of multivitamins in a suicide attempt, are anxious. They ask the nurse about what will be done for their son. The nurse correctly explains that their son's stomach will be washed and emptied of contents. This process is known as _____.

> **Answer:** Gastric lavage
>
> **Rationale:** Gastric lavage is commonly used to remove unwanted stomach contents.
>
> **Client Need:** Physiological Integrity

80.   A young child is admitted to the pediatric unit with a diagnosis of meningitis. The nurse knows the *priority* nursing intervention for this client is which of the following?

1. Administration of intravenous antibiotics as ordered.
2. Monitor vital signs every 4 hours as ordered.
3. Encourage fluids by mouth to decrease temperature.
4. Maintain the child on isolation precautions.

> **Answer:** 1
>
> **Rationale:** The priority is to administer the prescribed intravenous antibiotics as soon as the organism is identified. The other choices are important to do, but they are not the priority at this time.
>
> **Client Need:** Physiological Integrity

81.   The nurse is dining at a restaurant when a woman begins to scream that her husband is choking. The nurse's **initial** nursing action is to do which of the following?

1. Instruct the wife to call 911.
2. Ask the victim if he can speak.
3. Administer a back blow.
4. Administer an abdominal thrust.

Answer: 2

Rely on your knowledge of CPR.

Rationale: Before rescue efforts are put into place, the victim should be asked if he can speak. It is important that, if possible, he try to clear his own airway. Also, if he can speak he can move air. If necessary, someone other than the wife should be directed to call 911.

Client Need: Physiological Integrity

82. A 20-year-old male client is admitted to the hospital after falling off a ladder. He has suffered a head injury, and the physician suspects there may be cerebral anoxia. The nurse knows that an **early** sign of cerebral anoxia is which of the following?

1. Cyanosis.
2. Seizures.
3. Decreased intracranial pressure.
4. Restlessness.

Answer: 4

Rationale: Restlessness is an early indication of cerebral anoxia. Cyanosis is seen with hypoxia. Seizure activity is associated with increased intracranial pressure and can be a late sign and symptom of cerebral anoxia.

Client Need: Physiological Integrity

83. A 48-year-old married mother of three teenage children is diagnosed with infectious hepatitis A. The nurse is educating the client and her family in preventive techniques. The single **most important action** in the prevention of this disease is which of the following?

1. Do not frequent fast food establishments.
2. Avoid eating raw foods.
3. Establish good hand-washing habits.
4. Receive active immunization.

Answer: 3

Rationale: The most effective way of preventing this disease, as with most infectious diseases, is good hand-washing practices. It is not realistic to ask families to avoid eating out and to avoid all raw foods. Passive immunization is preventive.

> Did you remember hand washing, hand washing, hand washing?

Client Need: Health Promotion and Maintenance

---

84. A nurse is caring for a client with emphysema. When developing this client's plan of care, the nurse includes all of the following nursing interventions *except*

   1. Teach the client pursed lip breathing.
   2. Encourage the client to alternate activity with rest periods.
   3. Administer low flow oxygen by nasal cannula.
   4. Restrict fluid intake to less than 2000 ml per day.

Answer: 4

Rationale: It is important for the client with emphysema to learn pursed lip breathing, to alternate periods of activity with periods of rest, and to have low flow oxygen. It is inappropriate to restrict the client's fluid intake to 2000 ml per day. The client, unless contraindicated, should be encouraged to drink at least 3000 ml of fluid a day.

> Did you notice the word in *italics* in the stem?

Client Need: Physiological Integrity

---

85. The nurse is caring for a client with a hiatal hernia. The client complains of abdominal pain associated with eating. The nurse teaches the client recommended dietary changes for clients with hiatal hernia. Which statements, if made by the client, indicate that teaching was effective? Select all that apply.

1. "I will lie down for one half hour after meals."
2. "I will consume less caffeine and spicy foods."
3. "I will sleep with my head elevated onto pillows."
4. "I will try not to gain weight."

Answers: 2, 3, and 4

Rationale: It is important for the client with a hiatal hernia **not** to lie down after consuming food. It is good for the client to consume less caffeine and spicy foods, sleep with the head of the bed elevated, and try to maintain a stable weight.

Client Need: Physiological Integrity

---

86. A client comes to the emergency room after being hit in the right eye. The client's right eye is patched, and the client appears to be anxious. The nurse caring for this client knows to approach the client from which side?

_____

Answer: Left

Rationale: The nurse should approach the client from the left side so that the client is aware someone is approaching.

Client Need: Physiological Integrity

Ah-ha! Did you remember to stretch and deep breathe?

---

87. A 2-day postoperative client is ordered a full liquid diet. The nurse knows that all the following foods may be included on the client's tray *except*

1. Skim milk.
2. Ice cream.
3. Tomato juice.
4. Chicken broth.

Answer: 4

Rationale: Chicken broth is considered a clear liquid food item. Skim milk, ice cream, fruit and vegetable juices, puddings, and ice cream are considered full liquid food items.

Client Need: Physiological Integrity

88.   When assessing clients, nurses know it is important to include family members. What is the best way for the nurse to determine the members of a client's family?

1. Include people who live in the same house with the client.
2. Include people who are related to the client by blood and marriage.
3. Include people whom the client views as family.
4. Include people who you assess can adequately support the client.

Answer: 3

Rationale: It is not appropriate for the nurse to determine or guess who the members of a client's family are. The client should be the one to tell the nurse whom they view as family.

Client Need: Health Promotion and Maintenance

89.   The nurse admits an 85-year-old woman with Alzheimer's disease. The nurse notes that the client's 86-year-old spouse seems to be exhausted. He states that he is finding it more and more difficult to care for his wife. What is the nurse's *priority* intervention for this client and her spouse?

1. Recommend the husband place his wife in a long-term care facility.
2. Suggest the husband see a counselor to help cope with his exhaustion.
3. Encourage the husband to talk about his difficulties in caring for his wife.
4. Tell the husband he needs help immediately and insist he call a family meeting.

Answer: 3

Rationale: It is important for the nurse to encourage the husband to talk about his difficulties regarding caring for his wife. It is inappropriate for the nurse to recommend the husband place his wife in a long-term care facility. It is not the nurse's place to call a family meeting.

Client Need: Psychosocial Integrity

90.   A 6-month-old infant has had surgery to correct intussusception. The pediatrician has ordered clear liquids by mouth. The nurse correctly administers which of the following?

1. Oral electrolyte solution.
2. Half-strength infant formula.
3. Full-strength infant formula.
4. Sterile water.

Answer: 1

Rationale: Oral electrolyte solution is a better choice than sterile water. Any strength formula is considered a full liquid diet.

Client Need: Physiological Integrity

91.   A client is postbronchoscopy with biopsy. His vital signs are stable, and he is coughing up blood-tinged sputum. The nurse correctly documents this finding, which is known as _____.

Answer: Hemoptysis

Rationale: Hemoptysis is a common occurrence after bronchoscopy with biopsy. The signs and symptoms of hemorrhage must be watched for closely, such as frank bleeding.

Client Need: Physiological Integrity

92.   A client is admitted to your unit with severe dehydration. The physician orders fluid resuscitation and instructs the nurse to administer normal saline intravenously at 200 ml per hour for 8 hours. How many liters of fluid will the client receive during the nurse's 8-hour shift?

_____

> Did you remember *not* to label your answer? The label was included in the stem of the question.

Answer: 1.6

Rationale: If the client is to receive 200 ml per hour for 8 hours, the nurse multiplies 200 ml by 8 hours for a total of 1600 ml. One liter of intravenous fluid contains 1000 ml; therefore the total volume in liters of normal saline the client would receive in 8 hours is 1.6.

Client Need: Physiological Integrity

93.   The physician orders 125 mcg of digoxin every morning by mouth for his client. The pharmacy dispenses digoxin in 0.25 mg scored tablets. How many tablets should the nurse administer for one dose?

1. ½.
2. 1.
3. 1½.
4. 2.

> Did you remember *not* to label your answer? The label was included in the stem of the question.

Answer: 1

Rationale: The nurse begins by converting 125 mcg to 0.125 mg. The formula used is dose desired (0.125 mg) divided by the dose on hand (0.25 mg) and multiplied by the quantity on hand (1 tablet). The answer is ½ tablet.

Client Need: Physiological Integrity

94.   A nursing instructor is teaching a class of nursing students basic principles of health assessment. Mark the area on the following drawing where the nurse's hand should be placed to palpate the liver.

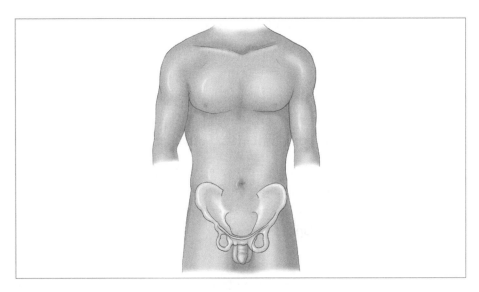

Answer: (The tester should mark the upper right quadrant of the abdomen with an "X.")

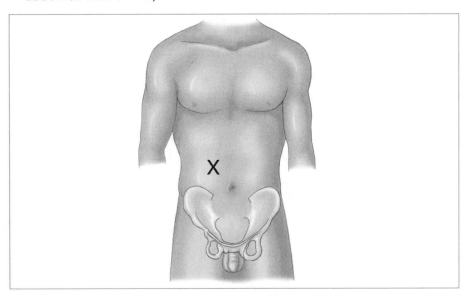

Rationale: The liver is palpated in the client's right upper quadrant. The nurse should stand on the client's right side and begin palpation to the right of midline. The fingers of the nurse's hand should point toward the client's head.

Client Need: Health Promotion and Maintenance

95. A pediatric advanced practice nurse is examining the ears of a child complaining of an earache. The nurse determines the client has otitis media. What physical finding would lead the nurse to make this diagnosis?

1. A pink and flat tympanic membrane.
2. A red and bulging tympanic membrane.
3. The absence of earwax.
4. An abundance of earwax.

Answer: 2

Rationale: In a child with otitis media the tympanic membrane appears red and bulging. A tympanic membrane that is pink and flat is normal. Earwax is typically not associated with otitis media.

Client Need: Physiological Integrity

96. A client has been diagnosed with deep vein thrombosis and has an intravenous infusion of heparin sodium infusing at 1000 units per hour. The concentration in the intravenous bag is 10,000 units in 500 ml. When completing the client intake and output sheet, how much should the nurse document as intake from this infusion in an 8-hour shift?

_____

> Did you remember to label your answer? The label was not included in the stem of the question.

Answer: 400 ml

Rationale: The nurse would use a ratio and proportion formula: 10,000 units is to 500 ml as 1000 units is to X ml. The answer is 50 ml per hour. This is multiplied by 8 hours, and the answer is 400 ml.

Client Need: Physiological Integrity

97. A client is being admitted to the cardiac care unit with a diagnosis of left ventricular myocardial infarction. The nurse knows that clients with left-sided heart failure usually present with which of the following symptoms? Select all that apply.

   1. Orthopnea.
   2. Abdominal pain.
   3. Dyspnea.
   4. Tachycardia.
   5. Hepatomegaly.

   Answers: 1, 3, and 4

   Rationale: Signs and symptoms of left-sided heart failure include dyspnea, crackles, tachycardia, orthopnea, and fatigue. Some clients experience nonproductive cough and hemoptysis.

   Client Need: Physiological Integrity

98. The nurse knows that when you are taking a client's apical pulse it is best to place the stethoscope over which part of the chest? Mark the following diagram with an "X."

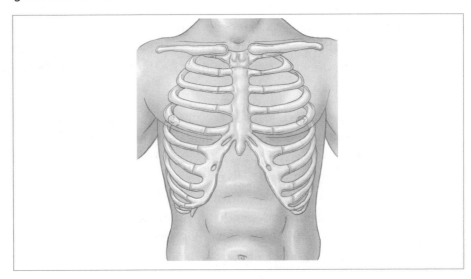

Answer: (The tester should mark the diagram at the left fifth intercostal space, mid-line.)

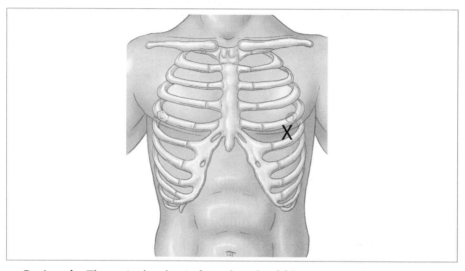

Rationale: The apical pulse is found at the fifth intercostal space, mid-line on the left chest.

Client Need: Physiological Integrity

99.   A client who has been diagnosed with terminal cancer is transferred to hospice care. A hospice nurse makes an initial visit to the client's home. Which information would be most important for the nurse to provide the client and the family members?

    1. Hospice care is focused on controlling symptoms, relieving pain, and providing the family with bereavement services.

    2. Hospice care is a multidisciplinary team that provides services based on the client's ability to pay.

    3. Hospice services are provided to clients in the comfort of their home and functions independently of physicians.

    4. Hospice services are best provided to the client and to the family members when care is given in a hospice facility.

Answer: 1

Rationale: Hospice care is focused on assisting the client to deal with symptoms and pain and to provide bereavement services to family members. Care is not based on the ability to pay. Hospice services are provided under the direction of a physician. Hospice care is also provided in the client's home.

Client Need: Physiological Integrity

100. It is recommended that all women over the age of 50 receive what annual diagnostic study?

_____

Answer: Mammography

Rationale: The American Cancer Society and the National Cancer Institute recommend annual mammography for women over the age of 50 to detect evidence of early breast cancer.

Client Need: Health Promotion and Maintenance

101. A client is 40 weeks gestation and is to have a fetal biophysical profile. The nurse knows that this evaluates fetal well-being. Which of the following components are included in a fetal biophysical profile? Select all that apply.

1. Fetal breathing.
2. Fetal motion.
3. Femur length.
4. Amniotic fluid index.
5. Nonstress test.

Answers: 1, 2, 4, and 5

Rationale: A fetal biophysical profile includes a nonstress test, fetal breathing, fetal motion, fetal tone, and amniotic fluid measurement.

Client Need: Physiological Integrity

102. Normal care for a newborn umbilical cord would include all the following interventions *except*

1. Washing the cord daily with mild soap and water.
2. Keeping the edge of the diaper below the cord.
3. Wiping the base of the cord two to three times a day.
4. Sponge bathing the newborn until the cord falls off.

Answer: 1

Rationale: Normal newborn cord care includes applying alcohol several times a day to help the cord dry. Sponge bathing the newborn and keeping the diaper below the level of the cord is recommended. The cord should not be washed.

Client Need: Safe Effective Care Environment

103. A female client is brought to the emergency department after being mugged and beaten. The client sits quietly and calmly in the examination room. The nurse caring for this client recognizes that this behavior is a protective mechanism known as which of the following?

1. Denial.
2. Displacement.
3. Redirection.
4. Disassociation.

Answer: 1

Rationale: Denial is a defensive coping mechanism used to protect the client from increased anxiety levels. The client consciously disowns intolerable thoughts and ideas. It is a common response in victims of violent crimes.

Client Need: Psychosocial Integrity

104. The nurse is caring for a client who has just had a cardiac catheterization. The nursing care plan for this client includes all the following nursing interventions **except**

1. Maintaining the client on bed rest.
2. Keeping the involved leg straight.
3. Elevating the head of the bed no more than 30 degrees.
4. Keeping the client NPO for 4 hours.

Answer: 4

Rationale: Clients who undergo cardiac catheterization should be maintained on bed rest with the involved leg straight to aid in clot formation. Elevation of the head should be limited to 30 degrees. The client does not have to be kept NPO and may eat after the procedure.

Client Need: Physiological Integrity

105. The nurse is preparing to palpate the uterine fundus of a client who is 22 weeks gestation. When measuring the fundal height, identify the area on the abdomen where the nurse would expect to feel the uterine fundus.

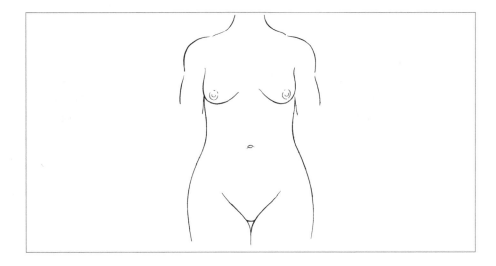

Answer: (At 22 weeks gestation, the fundal height should be just above the level of the umbilicus.)

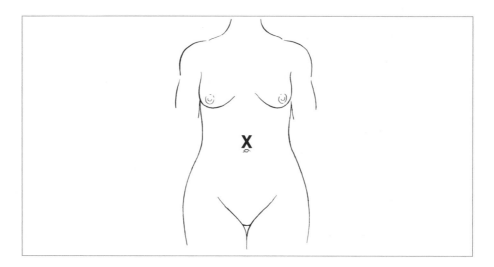

Rationale: Between 18 weeks gestation and approximately 34 weeks gestation the fundal height in centimeters is approximately equivalent to gestation age.

Client Need: Health Promotion and Maintenance

106. A postoperative client who had abdominal surgery 24 hours ago is out of bed sitting in a chair. The client suddenly complains of a pulling sensation and pain in his surgical incision. The nurse *assesses* the client's surgical wound and finds there has been an evisceration. What is the nurse's **priority** intervention?

  1. Immediately administer prescribed antibiotics intravenously.
  2. Assess the client for signs of shock.
  3. Cover the surgical wound with saline-soaked sterile dressings.
  4. Apply an abdominal binder.

Answer: 3

Rationale: When a postoperative surgical client experiences an evisceration, the priority nursing intervention is to cover the surgical wound with sterile saline-soaked dressings. The nurse should then notify the client's physician and prepare to transport the client to the operating room.

Client Need: Physiological Integrity

107. A client is admitted to your unit and is placed in an isolation room. The client's room is equipped with a glass thermometer. The nurse taking the client's oral temperature knows that the thermometer should remain under the client's tongue for a minimum of how many minutes?

1. 2 minutes.
2. 3 minutes.
3. 5 minutes.
4. 7 minutes.

Answer: 2

Rationale: Three minutes is the minimum amount of time needed to accurately measure a client's oral temperature using a glass thermometer.

Client Need: Physiological Integrity

108. A client admitted to the hospital with congestive heart failure has been taking Lasix to manage his condition. The nurse notes that the client has not been receiving supplemental electrolytes. The client had a full blood workup done in the morning. What laboratory value should the nurse assess before administering the Lasix?

1. Potassium.
2. Sodium.
3. Chloride.
4. Bicarbonate.

Answer: 1

Rationale: Lasix is a loop diuretic, which promotes excretion of potassium. The nurse should assess the client's potassium level before administering the Lasix to prevent hypokalemia.

Client Needs: Physiological Integrity

---

109. A client is admitted with type 1 diabetes mellitus. On afternoon rounds the nurse finds the client lying in bed, sweating, and complaining of lightheadedness and palpitations. The nurse assesses the client and finds that his pulse rate is tachycardic. What complication should the nurse suspect?

_____

Answer: Hypoglycemia

Rationale: The most common signs and symptoms of hypoglycemia include sweating, tachycardia, tremors, palpitations, and lightheadedness.

Client Need: Physiological Integrity

> Knowing the signs and symptoms of hypo- and hyperglycemia is a basic nursing requirement that you will need throughout your career.

---

110. The client is admitted to your unit with a diagnosis of chronic obstructive pulmonary disease. When performing a physical assessment on this client, you would expect the client's chest to be what shape?

1. Concave.
2. Convex.
3. Kyphotic.
4. Barrel.

Answer: 4

Rationale: Clients with chronic obstructive pulmonary disease chronically use accessory muscles to assist with respiratory effort. The chest wall eventually develops in an anterior-posterior diameter, making it appear barrel shaped.

Client Need: Physiological Integrity

111. A nurse is caring for a client who recently underwent surgery for insertion of a permanent pacemaker. Which of the following orders, if written by the client's physician, should the nurse question?

1. Serum blood levels for cardiac enzymes in the morning.
2. Magnetic resonance imaging of the chest.
3. Begin physical therapy.
4. Regular low-sodium diet.

Answer: 2

Rationale: Clients with pacemakers should not be scheduled for magnetic resonance imaging. The magnets in the machine could dislodge the internal pacemaker.

Client Need: Physiological Integrity

112. A woman who is 18 weeks pregnant comes to the clinic for her monthly assessment. The client tells the nurse that she felt light fluttering in her stomach yesterday. The nurse correctly explains to the client that this is normal and is known as

_____

Answer: Quickening

Rationale: Quickening is often described as fluttering by clients between 16 and 22 weeks gestation. It is caused by fetal movement and is classified as a presumptive sign of pregnancy.

Client Need: Health Promotion and Maintenance

113. The nursery nurse is preparing to administer vitamin K (AquaMEPHYTON) by intramuscular injection to a newborn. The nurse knows the primary muscle for intramuscular injections in infants is which of the following?

1. Vastus lateralis.
2. Ventrogluteal muscle.
3. Dorsogluteal muscle.
4. Deltoid muscle.

Answer: 1

Rationale: The vastus lateralis is the preferred site for intramuscular injections in infants. Therefore answers 2, 3, and 4 are incorrect.

Client Need: Physiological Integrity

114. A pediatric client has amoxicillin 350 mg by mouth ordered four times a day. The vial reads amoxicillin 250 mg per 5 ml. How many milliliters should the nurse administer for each dose?

_____

Answer: 7

Rationale: The formula used is calculating drug dosages. The desired dose is 350 mg divided by 250 mg and multiplied by 5 ml. The answer is 7 milliliters.

> Did you remember *not* to label your answer? The label was included in the stem of the question.

Client Need: Physiological Integrity

115. The nurse knows that the uterus in postpartum clients progressively returns to a prepregnancy or nonpregnancy state. This process is known as _____.

Answer: Involution

Rationale: Involution is the return of the woman's body in the postpartum period to a state of prepregnancy. It involves the shrinking and repositioning of the uterus, and lasts for approximately 6 weeks.

Client Need: Health Promotion and Maintenance

116. A pediatric client is admitted to your unit with a diagnosis of Wilms' tumor. In which anatomical structure is a Wilms' tumor located?

1. Liver.
2. Kidney.
3. Pancreas.
4. Spleen.

Answer: 2

Rationale: Wilms' tumor, also known as nephroblastoma, is located in the kidney. It is the most common tumor of childhood.

Client Need: Physiological Integrity

117. A client comes to the psychiatric emergency room and tells the nurse of his plan for committing suicide. After discussing the plan with a psychiatrist, the client agrees to a voluntary admission to the psychiatric unit. The client asks the nurse, "How long do I have to stay in the hospital?" What is an appropriate response for the nurse to make?

1. "You may leave the hospital when you want as long as you are not suicidal."
2. "Your doctor is the only one who can discharge you."
3. "There will be a court hearing to decide that question."
4. "You must stay for a minimum of 7 days."

Answer: 1

Rationale: A person who voluntarily admits themselves to a psychiatric hospital may sign out of the hospital at any time, unless the health care team determines the client is suicidal and/or homicidal. The client's physician can also write a discharge order. There will be no court hearing, and there is no minimum stay.

> Did you choose answer 1 because it is the most comprehensive answer?

Client Need: Psychosocial Integrity

118. A newly delivered infant is admitted to the newborn nursery. On physical examination, the nurse includes measurement of the infant's chest circumference. Identify the anatomical landmark the nurse uses to correctly perform this assessment.

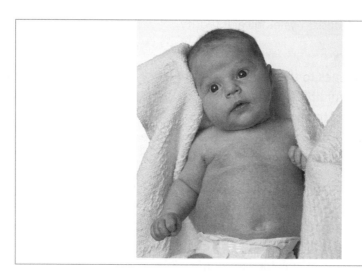

Answer: (The infants nipple line.)

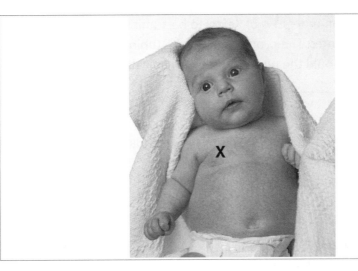

Rationale: Chest circumference is most accurately measured when the nurse places the measuring tape around the newborn's chest with the tape covering the nipples.

Client Need: Health Promotion and Maintenance

---

119.   A nurse is attending a cardiopulmonary resuscitation (CPR) class. When learning infant CPR, the nurse knows that which of the following is the anatomical area where the pulse is assessed?

1. Radial.
2. Femoral.
3. Carotid.
4. Brachial.

Answer: 4

Rationale: The brachial pulse is the preferred site for assessing the infant heart rate during CPR. The carotid pulse is used to assess the heart rate in children and adults.

Client Need: Physiological Integrity

120. A physician orders 1 g of Kefzol to be administered in 50 ml of normal saline in 20 minutes. The drop factor on the tubing is 20. In how many drops per minute should the nurse infuse the medication?

_____

Answer: 50

Rationale: The correct formula is a standard intravenous formula. The 50 ml (volume) is divided by 20 minutes (time) and multiplied by 20 (drop factor). The correct answer is 50 drops per minute.

> Did you remember *not* to label your answer? The label was part of the stem of the question.

Client Need: Physiological Integrity

121. A woman in labor is asking the nurse about the equipment used in the labor room. She is particularly interested in the instrument used to locate her baby's heart rate. The nurse correctly informs the client that this instrument is known as a _____.

Answer: Fetal heart rate transducer

Rationale: A fetal heart rate transducer is used with conducting gel and placed over the part of the fetus, usually the back, where the heart rate can be heard best.

Client Need: Safe Effective Care Environment

122. A mother tells the pediatric nurse that her toddler drinks a quart of milk a day and has a poor appetite for solid foods. The nurse knows this pediatric client is at risk for which of the following?

1. Iron deficiency anemia.
2. Protein overload.
3. Faulty carbohydrate metabolism.
4. Obesity.

Answer: 1

Rationale: Toddlers who drink milk and skip meals are often at risk for developing iron deficiency anemia. Protein overload is associated with renal disease. Faulty carbohydrate metabolism is associated with diabetes. The child is not at risk for obesity.

Client Need: Health Promotion and Maintenance

123. A nurse prepares an intravenous solution of 1000 ml of D_5W with 48 units of regular insulin. The infusion is to run at 2 units per hour. The nurse uses microtubing. The nurse should set the infusion pump at how many drops per minute?

_____

Answer: 42

Rationale: A ratio and proportion formula is used to calculate the answer. 48 units is to 1000 ml as 2 units is to *X* milliliters. The answer is 41.6 or 42 drops per minute.

Client Need: Physiological Integrity

> Did you label your answer? The question this time indicated the dosing label so you should not have labeled your answer.

124. A term primipara is admitted to the labor and delivery unit. She is having uterine contractions every 3 minutes lasting 50 to 60 seconds. On vaginal examination the nurse determines the client is 6 cm dilated and 100% effaced. Her temperature is 98.6°F, pulse 88, and blood pressure 84/40. What is the nurse's **priority** action?

1. Document the findings as normal.
2. Position the client for comfort.
3. Prepare for an immediate vaginal delivery.
4. Turn the client on her left side.

Answer: 4

Rationale: Decreasing pressure on the inferior vena cava will help raise the client's blood pressure. The nurse should then recheck the blood pressure and notify the obstetrician if the intervention is not effective.

Client Need: Physiological Integrity

---

125.   A nurse is assigned to care for a client whose cultural background is unfamiliar. All the following nursing interventions are appropriate when caring for a client from a different culture **except**

1. Explain the nurse's cultural beliefs to the client.
2. Respect the client's cultural beliefs.
3. Ask the client what cultural requirements should be included in the plan of care.
4. Understand that different cultures define health and wellness in different ways.

Answer: 1

Rationale: The nurse should never impose his or her cultural or religious beliefs on a client. It is important for nurses to respect the client's cultural beliefs, to include these cultural beliefs in the client's plan of care, and to understand and accept differences within cultures.

Client Need: Psychosocial Integrity

---

126.   An infant is brought to the well-baby clinic for a 2-month checkup. The physician tells the mother he is assessing for Ortolani's sign. The nurse knows this assessment is for dislocation of which of the following joints?

1. Hip.
2. Knee.
3. Shoulder.
4. Elbow.

Answer: 1

Rationale: Ortolani's sign is assessed when the infant's hips are abducted while flexing the infant's knees. The pediatrician listens for a clicking sound as the femoral head enters the acetabulum. This finding indicates a congenital dislocated hip.

Client Need: Health Promotion and Maintenance

127. A 65-year-old client returns to his room from the postanesthesia care unit. The physician orders 1 l of D5 ½ normal saline to infuse at 100 ml per hour. The nurse is using microtubing. At what rate will the nurse administer the intravenous solution in drops per minute?

1. 25.
2. 60.
3. 125.
4. 100.

Answer: 4

Rationale: The flow rate of 100 ml per hour would be divided by 60 minutes and then multiplied by the drop factor. Microtubing has a drop factor of 60. The answer is 100 drops per minute.

Client Need: Physiological Integrity

Did you remember that microtubing has a drop factor of 60 and when using microtubing the drops per minute *equal* the milliliters per hour?

1. The delivery room nurse notes that 5 minutes after birth a newborn has a pink trunk and head, bluish hands and feet, and flexed extremities. Also, the infant has a soft cry, a heart rate of 130, and abdominal respirations of 40. The nurse would correctly assign which Apgar score?

APGAR SCORE			
Sign	0	1	2
Heart rate (bpm)	Absent	Slow (< 100)	≥ 100
Respirations	Absent	Slow, irregular	Good, crying
Muscle tone	Limp	Some flexion	Active motion
Reflex irritability (catheter in nares, tactile stimulation)	No response	Grimace	Cough, sneeze, cry
Color	Blue or pale	Pink body with blue extremities	Completely pink

Answer: 8

Rationale: The neonate earns two points each for the heart rate, respiratory rate, and muscle tone. The weak cry and acrocyanosis of the hands and feet earn one point each for a total of eight points.

Client Need: Physiological Integrity

2. A client with angina comes to the emergency room. He tells the nurse he took his daily medications that morning, including 3 nitroglycerine tablets sublingually just before coming to the hospital. Which of the following signs and symptoms should the nurse expect the client to exhibit? Select all that apply.

1. Tightness in the chest.
2. General muscle cramping.
3. Pressure on the chest.
4. Jaw pain.
5. Bradypnea.
6. Bradycardia.

Answers: 1, 3, and 4

Rationale: A patent with angina frequently complains of tightness in the chest, chest pressure, and jaw pain. General muscle cramping is not associated with angina. Bradypnea and bradycardia are also not associated with angina.

> Remember to concentrate on information included in the stem of the question that is directly connected to the answer options.

Client Need: Physiological Integrity

---

3.   A newly delivered mother has decided to breastfeed her newborn baby. Which statement by the mother indicates to the nurse that diet teaching for the breastfeeding mother has been successful?

 1. "I will decrease roughage and increase carbohydrates at each meal."
 2. "I will restrict the amount of salt that I take in my diet."
 3. "I will increase the amount of calcium and protein at each meal."
 4. "I will increase fats and carbohydrates at dinner."

Answer: 3

Rationale: A breastfeeding mother should increase calcium and protein in her diet. The production of breastmilk places demands on the mother's resources for both of these nutrients. She should be encouraged to include milk, cheese, and spinach in her diet. Answer 1, 2, and 4 are not necessary changes for the breastfeeding mother.

Client Need: Health Promotion and Maintenance

---

4.   A 56-year-old client with type 1 diabetes is discussing care at home with the nurse. The client states that he understands the importance of proper foot care. The nurse further questions the client and discovers the client is very knowledgeable regarding diabetic foot care. Which comment by the client leads the nurse to believe the client understands the teaching?

1. "I will use iodine on any injuries to my feet."
2. "I will use cream on my feet, especially between my toes."
3. "I will check my feet every day for sores and bruises."
4. "I will soak my feet in salt water every night before going to bed."

Answer: 3

Rationale: The client with type 1 diabetes should check his or her feet on a daily basis. He or she should not use iodine because it is irritating to skin. Diabetics should also never use cream in between the toes. Soaking in salt water is not recommended.

> Did you remember to try 1 B and 3 Gs for this teaching question?

Client Need: Health Promotion and Maintenance

5. A woman who is in her first trimester is being assessed at a prenatal visit. Which of the following statements, if made by the client, is consistent for a woman in the first trimester of pregnancy? Select all that apply.

1. "My husband told me we will have to buy a larger car and not drive our two-seater sports car any longer."
2. "I can't believe this pregnancy happened to me. I'm not sure how it happened."
3. "I hope the baby has blonde hair and blue eyes like the rest of my family members."
4. "I used lot's of pink and blue and yellow and green striped wall paper for decorating the baby's room."
5. "I hope I don't get too fat and have to wear the maternity clothes too soon."
6. "My husband and I are going this weekend to buy a crib and furniture for the baby's room."

Answers: 1, 2, and 5

Rationale: A woman in the first trimester of pregnancy is ambivalent about the pregnancy. Decorating and shopping, along with imagining what her baby will look like, are more common in the second and third trimesters.

Client Need: Psychosocial Integrity

6. A student nurse is caring for a client with a serious skin infection. The client is using topical gentamycin sulfate. Which of the following statements, if made by the client, indicates to the nurse a need for additional teaching?

   1. "I no longer will go out and suntan for long hours."
   2. "Once the area is healed I will stop applying the ointment."
   3. "I will notify my doctor if the infection looks worse."
   4. "I should apply the cream to large areas around the infection and to all open areas."

Answer: 4

Rationale: It is not recommended to apply antibiotic cream to large areas surrounding the infection nor directly into open areas.

> Did you try to use Bs and Gs? This is clearly a question where goods and bads would be helpful.

Client Need: Physiological Integrity

7. A middle-aged male client suffered a myocardial infarction 4 days ago. He has recovered nicely with no further episodes of chest pain. The physician has ordered a gradual increase in the client's activity level. Which priority assessment should the nurse make to determine that the client's activity level is inappropriate?

   1. Decreased edema of the lower extremities.
   2. Increased dyspnea when transferring from bed to chair.
   3. Decreased appetite.
   4. Weight loss.

Answer: 2

Rationale: The client should not experience increased dyspnea when transferring from the bed to the chair. The decreased edema is a good sign. Decreased appetite and weight loss are not associated with activity.

Client Need: Physiological Integrity

8. A 2-year-old toddler is admitted to the pediatric unit. The mother reports a history of abdominal pain, vomiting, diarrhea, and anorexia. The nurse correctly suspects the child has plumbism, which is also known as _____.

Answer: Lead poisoning

Rationale: Children who ingest or inhale toxins, such as lead, become very ill and need adequate treatment.

Client Need: Physiological Integrity

9. A 45-year-old client has just been diagnosed with type 2 diabetes mellitus. She asks the nurse what she needs to do to take care of herself. The nurse prepares a teaching plan for the client that includes which of the following as the **first** step in the nursing process?

1. Establish short-term realistic goals for the client.
2. Implement the use of a teaching video and provide brochure material to aid in the education process.
3. Assess what the client knows about caring for herself and managing her diabetes.
4. Evaluate the effectiveness of the client's admission teaching plan.

Answer: 3

Rationale: Assessment is the first step of the nursing process. Once the nurse assesses the client, goals can be established and

Did you remember to **Assess Before Caring?**

interventions put into action. The last step is to evaluate if the goals for the client have been met.

Client Need: Health Promotion and Maintenance

10. A 49-year-old client comes to the emergency department with nonspecific complaints. He states that he just does not feel like himself. Screening blood work is drawn, and it is discovered the client has a low potassium level. The emergency room nurse anticipates which of the following physiological responses related to the client's hypokalemia? The client is at risk for developing

1. Cardiac arrhythmias.
2. Hypoglycemia.
3. Bradypnea.
4. Increased appetite.

Answer: 1

Rationale: Potassium levels are directly related to cardiac function. A low level can cause irregular heart rates. Answers 2, 3, and 4 are not related to low potassium levels.

Client Need: Physiological Integrity

11. The nursing supervisor is teaching a class of newly hired unlicensed assistive personnel. The supervisor is emphasizing the importance of hand washing in the prevention of the spread of germs and should include which of the following statements?

1. "If you're going to wear gloves, you do not have to wash your hands."
2. "Hand washing has been proven to be the best method in preventing the spread of germs."
3. "Waterless commercial products are ineffective in killing bacteria and microorganisms."
4. "The hands are not typically considered a source of infection."

Answer: 2

Rationale: Research has shown that proper hand washing is the best method in the prevention of the spread of infection. It is important to wash hands after removing gloves. Water-less products have been effective in controlling germs. The hands are a primary source of infection.

Did you remember to promote hand washing, hand washing, hand washing?

Client Need: Safe Effective Care Environment

12.   A postoperative client is receiving intravenous fluids and is to receive a unit of whole blood. The nurse is to observe for signs and symptoms of circulatory overload. Which nursing assessment is the *priority* in the early detection of circulatory overload?

1. The quality of the client's skin turgor.
2. The character of the client's respirations.
3. Measurement of the client's intake and output.
4. Changes in the client's blood pressure.

Answer: 2

Rationale: One of the earliest indications of circulatory overload is a change in the character of the client's respirations. Other major signs and symptoms include weight

Did you remember Airway, Breathing, Circulation?

gain, edema, puffiness of the eyes, distention of neck veins, and pulmonary edema. Answers 1, 3, and 4 have no direct relationship to circulatory overload.

Client Need: Health Promotion and Maintenance

13.   A healthcare practitioner who provides clients with incorrect or negligent treatment might be found guilty in a court of law of _____.

> **Answer:** Malpractice
>
> **Rationale:** Any health care provider who incorrectly cares for clients can be sued for malpractice.
>
> **Client Need:** Safe Effective Care Environment

14.   A newly admitted client at 38 weeks gestation has been diagnosed with severe preeclampsia. When completing the admission assessment for the client, the nurse should be alert for which of the following?

1. Tachycardia.
2. An elevated temperature.
3. Polyuria.
4. Complaints of headache and blurred vision.

> **Answer:** 4
>
> **Rationale:** A nurse monitoring clients with preeclampsia should assess for symptoms that include headache, blurred vision, excitability, nausea, and vomiting. Hypertension, proteinuria, and edema are the three classic signs of preeclampsia. Answers 1, 2, and 3 are not characteristic symptoms of preeclampsia.
>
> **Client Need:** Health Promotion and Maintenance

15.   The nurse knows that a priority goal in caring for a preterm infant is conservation of energy. Which nursing intervention **best** promotes conservation of energy?

1. Place elbow restraints on the newborn.
2. Change the infant's position every 2 hours.
3. Clustering activities.
4. Gavage feeding the preterm infant.

Answer: 3

Rationale: By clustering activities and organizing care, the nurse prevents excessive interruptions and allows the infant extended periods of rest. Restraints are not required and interfere with hand to mouth consoling behaviors. Changing of the infant's position is included in clustering activities. Gavage feeding is also included in clustering activities.

> **Did you use step 5 to answer this question?**

Client Need: Physiological Integrity

---

16.   A nurse is caring for a client who is postoperative. The client has had a cholecystectomy and is complaining of pain. Which of the following actions should the nurse take? Select all that apply.

   1. Offer the client a back rub.
   2. Medicate the client with the prescribed analgesic.
   3. Assess the client's pain level on a scale from 1 to 10.
   4. Notify the surgeon.
   5. Change the client's position.

Answers: 1, 2, 3, and 5

Rationale: Nonpharmacological remedies are often helpful is diminishing a client's pain. Properly assessing the pain and giving appropriate medication are important. There is no indication that the surgeon needs to be notified.

Client Need: Physiological Integrity

---

17.   An 85-year-old client has just had surgery. The physician orders Demerol (meperidine hydrochloride) 30 mg intramuscularly every 4 hours as needed. The label on the syringe reads 50 mg per 3 ml. How many milliliters should the nurse discard?

_____

Answer: 1.2

Rationale: The doctor ordered 30 mg. When 30 mg is divided by 50 mg × 3 ml, the answer is 1.8 ml. This is the amount to administer. When 1.8 is subtracted from 3, the remainder is 1.2. The amount of medication to be wasted is 1.2 ml.

> **Did you read the question correctly and calculate the amount of medication to discard?**

Client Need: Physiological Integrity.

---

18. A woman at 10 weeks gestation has been admitted complaining of abdominal pain and moderate vaginal bleeding. A diagnosis of suspected incomplete abortion is made. Which action by the nurse is **most** appropriate to include in the client's nursing care plan?

1. Keep the client NPO.
2. Assess and document the amount and type of vaginal bleeding.
3. Instruct the client in appropriate birth control methods.
4. Place the client on bed rest.

Answer: 2

Rationale: Assessment of the amount and type of vaginal bleeding should be included in the client's plan of care. Bleeding may continue until all of the products of conception have been expelled. It is important for the nurse to note the number of pads used and the amount and type of bleeding. There is no need to keep the client NPO and no indication the client requires birth control teaching. The client's activity level will be ordered by the physician.

> **Did you remember nurses Assess Before Caring?**

Client Need: Physiological Integrity

19.   The nurse is assessing the peripheral pulses of a newly admitted cardiac client. Identify the area in the figure where the nurse would palpate the left pedal pulse.

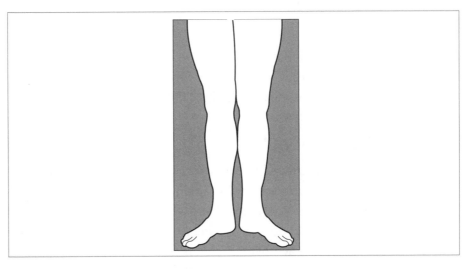

Answer: (The "X" would appear on the top of the foot)

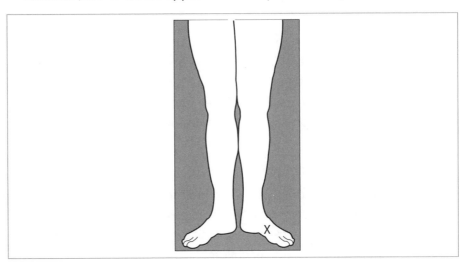

Rationale: The pedal pulse is located on the top of the foot.

Client Need: Physiological Integrity

20.   A nursing home nurse enters the day room and finds the window curtains on fire. Clients are panicking and the room is filling with smoke. The nurse acts quickly and performs all the following actions. Number the nursing actions in the priority order the nurse would complete them.

___ Close the door.
___ Sound the fire alarm.
___ Remove the residents from the room.
___ Document the nurse's observations.
___ Extinguish the fire.

Answer: 3, 2, 1, 5, 4

Rationale: The nurse's priority action is to remove the residents from danger. The nurse would then sound the fire alarm and close the door to contain the fire. If able, the nurse would extinguish the fire. The last thing the nurse would do is to document the occurrence on an incident report. Remember the acronym "RACE": rescue, alarm, confine, and extinguish.

Client Need: Safe Effective Care Environment

21.   A female client is brought to the mental health emergency room and states she has not been able to leave her home for weeks. She tells you she feels overwhelmed. The nurse further discovers that the client has lost her job and has not visited her children in their homes for months. What diagnosis would you expect the physician to place in the client's chart?

_____

Answer: Agoraphobia

Rationale: Agoraphobia is an irrational fear of leaving one's home. Usually, the client knows the fear is unreasonable. The diagnosis is further supported by the extreme results of the client's behavior such as loss of her job and not seeing her children.

Client Need: Psychosocial Integrity

22.   A school nurse is completing routine annual assessments on students entering high school. Assessment screening of the spine is included. The nurse examines a young athlete and detects an abnormal curvature of the spine. What diagnosis should the nurse suspect?

_____

Answer: Scoliosis

Rationale: Scoliosis is an abnormal lateral curvature of the spine found most often in children over the age of 10 years.

Client Need: Health Promotion and Maintenance

23.   The nurse is assigned to administer digoxin to a cardiac client. To correctly assess the apical pulse, mark the location on the following figure where the nurse would place the stethoscope.

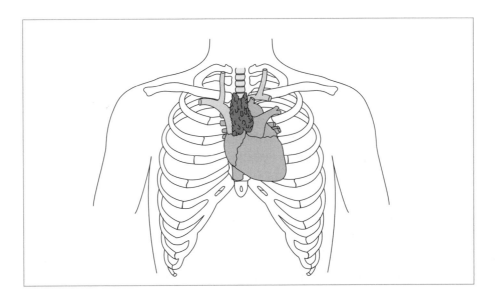

Answer: (left fifth intercostal space, midline)

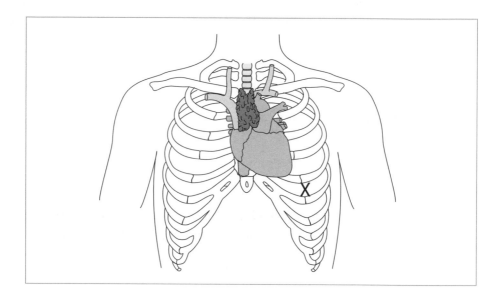

Rationale: The apical pulse is best heard at the left fifth intercostal space, midline

Client Need: Physiological Integrity

24. A preschool-aged child is brought to the clinic and diagnosed with Wilms' tumor. The nurse knows Wilms' tumors occur in young pediatric clients and are most commonly found in which organ?

Answer: Kidney

Rationale: Wilms' tumors, also known as nephroblastomas, are found in the kidney and usually are seen in children between the ages of 2 to 4 years.

Client Need: Physiological Integrity

25.   A client comes to the clinic at 23 weeks gestation for an amniocentesis. You inform the client that before the amniocentesis she should

1. Refrain from eating breakfast.
2. Give herself a fleet enema.
3. Empty her bladder.
4. Washed her abdomen with Betadine.

Answer: 3

Rationale: Emptying her bladder before amniocentesis prevents possible puncture of the bladder and displacement of the uterus and fetus. It is not necessary to fast for amniocentesis. It is also not necessary to have an enema. The nurse will cleanse the abdomen before the amniocentesis.

Client Need: Safe Effective Care Environment

26.   A 5-year-old comes to your unit after a tonsillectomy. The physician has ordered a clear liquid diet for the child. Which items should the nurse include on the child's lunch tray? Select all that apply.

1. Broth.
2. Apple juice.
3. Milk.
4. Ice cream.
5. Toast.
6. Lemon gelatin.

Answers: 1, 2, and 6

Rationale: Milk and ice cream are included in a full liquid diet. Broth, apple juice, and gelatin are included in a clear liquid diet.

Client Need: Physiological Integrity

27. A preschooler has been admitted to the hospital. The child is crying and reaching for her mother. What *actions* by the parents demonstrate an understanding of anxiety-reducing behaviors for their child?

 1. Scolding the child.
 2. Holding the child.
 3. Giving the child a toy to play with.
 4. Sitting next to the child's bedside.

Answer: 2

Rationale: It is recommended that the mother be allowed to hold and comfort the child.

Client Need: Psychosocial Integrity

28. A group of nurses are taking a class on infant resuscitation. The instructor stresses which of the following techniques for reviving an infant? Select all that apply.

 1. Hyperextend the head to open the infant's airway.
 2. Breathe only into the mouth of the infant.
 3. Use the brachial artery to check the infant's pulse.
 4. Use the tips of two fingers to compress the chest.
 5. Compress the infant's sternum ½ to 1 inch.

Answers: 3, 4, and 5

Rationale: When performing cardiopulmonary resuscitation on the infant, the rescuers should breathe into the mouth and nostrils of the infant. The brachial artery is the site of choice for pulse assessment. It is recommended that the tips of two fingers be used to compress the chest ½ to 1 inch.

Client Need: Physiological Integrity

29.   A nurse is admitting a client and is having trouble reading the physician's admission orders. What is the nurse's **best** action?

1. Clarify the order with another nurse.
2. Call the pharmacist to help interpret the physicians order.
3. Clarify the order with the physician.
4. Call the nursing supervisor for clarification.

Answer: 3

Rationale: Illegible writing can cause numerous errors, including medication errors. The admitting physician should clarify the orders. Interpretation by others could lead to a mistake.

Ah-ha! Did you remember to stretch and deep breathe?

Client Need: Safe Effective Care Environment

30.   A nurse is giving a new mother discharge instructions regarding circumcision care. The nurse knows that teaching was successful when the mother states which of the following? Select all that apply.

1. "I will allow 1 to 2 weeks for complete healing."
2. "I will apply petroleum jelly to the penis every time I change the baby's diaper."
3. "I know my baby must urinate before I can go home."
4. "I will call the doctor if I see any bleeding."
5. "I will soak the baby in a tub of warm water to help promote healing."

Answers: 2, 3, and 4

Rationale: Circumcision typically heals in 2 to 4 days. Infants cannot soak in a tub while the cord dries and falls off, in usually 10 to 14 days. The infant must void before being discharged. Bleeding must be reported immediately.

Client Need: Safe Effective Care Environment

31. A nurse is preparing to administer a unit of red blood cells. After verifying the order with another nurse, the primary nurse should verify the information on the blood label with the information on which of the following?

    1. The client's chart.

    2. The client's order sheet.

    3. The medication administration record.

    4. The client's wristband and in the presence of a second nurse.

Answer: 4

Rationale: It is general policy that two nurses verify the client's name and verify data with the client's wristband.

Did you look for the most comprehensive answer?

Client Need: Physiological Integrity

32. A new mother has had a spontaneous delivery without complications. She tells the nurse she wants to breastfeed. When the infant is brought in for the first breastfeeding, the client asks the nurse how much of the nipple should be put into the baby's mouth. Which of the following statements made by the nurse gives the client the *best* information?

    1. "You should place your nipple and some of the dark area around your nipple into the baby's mouth."

    2. "Babies know instinctively exactly how much of the nipple to take into the mouth."

    3. "Your baby's mouth is rather small so the baby will only take part of the nipple."

    4. "Your baby will nurse well when only the nipple is in the mouth."

Answer: 1

Rationale: Placing the nipple and part of the areola into the baby's mouth will aid in adequately compressing the milk ducts. This placement also decreases stress on the nipple and helps to prevent cracking and soreness.

Babies do not instinctively know how much of the nipple to take into the mouth. Regardless of the size of the baby's mouth, it is necessary for the baby to have the nipple and part of the areola in the mouth. It is never acceptable to have just the nipple in the baby's mouth.

Did you choose the most comprehensive answer for this question?

Client Need: Health Promotion and Maintenance

---

33. A client is to have an elective surgical procedure. When admitting the client, the nurse checks the surgical consent. The nurse understands the person legally responsible for obtaining the surgical consent is

1. The nurse.
2. The surgeon.
3. The unit clerk.
4. The anesthesiologist.

Answer: 2

Rationale: It is general policy that the person performing the procedure is responsible for obtaining the consent. This process includes explaining all aspects of the procedure to the client and answering all questions.

Client Needs: Safe Effective Care Environment

---

34. An elderly client is dying and requests to go home and be with her family. The family members want to bring the client home and inquire about hospice care. The nurse correctly informs the family members that hospice care

1. Will send only registered nurses to the home to care for the client.
2. Will direct care exclusively to the dying client.
3. Will attempt to extend the clients life as long as possible.
4. Will focus on the needs of the client and the family.

Answer: 4

Rationale: Supportive care is aimed at the client and family members. Prolonging life and using only registered nurses is not part of hospice care. Rather, hospice care utilizes the services of many resources.

Client Need: Physiological Integrity

---

35. A term used for the fertilized ovum is _____.

Answer: Zygote

Rationale: A zygote is the result of the union of two gametes.

Client Need: Physiological Integrity

---

36. A client is in need of increased protein intake. When selecting food items from the menu for the next day's meals, the nurse assists the client in appropriately choosing all the following items **except**

1. Yogurt.
2. Low-fat cheese.
3. Bacon.
4. Cooked beans.

Answer: 3

Rationale: All the items are sources of protein, but bacon is also high in fat and should be eaten in limited amounts for a healthy diet.

Client Need: Physiological Integrity

---

37. A client with angina pectoris is to be instructed on the proper way of taking nitroglycerin tablets sublingually. The nurse knows that teaching was effective when the client states which of the following?

1. "I will dial 911 after three nitroglycerin tablets taken every 5 minutes do not relieve my pain."
2. "I will dial 911 after taking four nitroglycerin tablets over a 20-minute period."
3. "I will call 911 when I have pain and then take the nitroglycerin tablets."
4. "I will drive myself to the emergency room if three tablets of nitroglycerin do not relieve my pain."

Answer: 1

Rationale: Nitroglycerin tablets should be taken every 5 minutes for three doses before calling 911. Calling 911 before taking the tablets is incorrect. Client's who do not get relief from nitroglycerin sublingually should never drive themselves to the hospital. The client should never take four tablets.

Did you use "good" and "bad" for this teaching question?

Client Need: Physiological Integrity

38. A client comes to the psychiatric emergency room and states that he and his family would be better off if he was dead. The *priority* response by the nurse is which of the following?

1. "Do you really think your family would be better off without you?"
2. "Are you thinking of killing yourself?"
3. "A day's rest will help you to think with a clearer mind."
4. "When did you first start feeling this way?"

Answer: 2

Rationale: It is crucial that a depressed client who verbalizes a death wish be asked directly about thoughts of suicide. Any other information would not be the priority.

Remember, safety is priority for the client.

Client Need: Psychosocial Integrity

39.   A nurse is caring for a multigravid client in active labor. The client is 7 cm dilated and 100% effaced. The fetus is at 1+ station, and the membranes are intact. The client suddenly states she needs to push. What is the nurse's *next* action?

1. Assist the client into a comfortable position to push.
2. Assess the perineum for signs of crowning.
3. Have the client pant during the next few contractions.
4. Tell the client not to push and help her to the bathroom to empty her bladder.

Answer: 3

Rationale: Panting has been known to ease the urge to push during contractions. The client is only 7 cm dilated and pushing prematurely causes edema and trauma. There is no evidence of crowning.

Client Need: Health Promotion and Maintenance

40.   A postoperative client is recovering nicely. Which of the following foods would the nurse encourage the client to select from the food menu to aid in the healing of the surgical wound?

1. A bacon, egg, and cheese sandwich.
2. Chicken and orange slices.
3. Green tea and a cheeseburger.
4. A pork chop and buttered noodles.

Answer: 2

Rationale: Protein and vitamin C are essential in promoting wound healing. Carbohydrates and fats should be taken in moderation.

Client Need: Physiological Integrity

Did you remember to choose chicken as a nutritionally valuable food?

41.   A newborn is found to have an apical pulse rate of 130 beats per minute. The nursery nurse should do which of the following?

1. Ask another nurse to verify the heart rate.
2. Document this as a normal finding.
3. Call the neonatologist to assess the newborn.
4. Prepare the newborn for transport to the neonatal intensive care unit.

Answer: 2

Rationale: The normal newborn heart rate is 120 to 160 beats per minute. The nurse should document the finding as normal. There is no need to verify the heart rate, call the neonatologist, or prepare to transport the newborn.

Client Need: Health Promotion and Maintenance

42.   A nurse is caring for an elderly client who just underwent a cardiac catheterization. Which priority nursing interventions should be included in the client's plan of care for the next 8 hours? Select all that apply.

1. Maintain pressure over the femoral puncture site.
2. Place the client in high Fowler's position.
3. Assess the femoral dressing for drainage and bleeding.
4. Monitor the client's vital signs every 4 hours and document.
5. Keep the client's hip and leg extended.
6. Allow the client bathroom privileges.

Answers: 1, 3, and 5

Rationale: Maintaining pressure over the puncture site prevents bleeding and promotes clot formation. Vital signs should be assessed every 15 minutes for the first hour and every 30 minutes for the second hour. Vital signs should then be assesses every hour for the next 4 hours. Assessing the dressing frequently will alert the nurse to bleeding. Preventing the leg and hip from flexing helps promote clot formation.

Client Need: Physiological Integrity

43. A toddler has been diagnosed with iron deficient anemia. The nurse instructs the mother to increase iron in the child's diet by including which of the following foods?

   1. Green squash and milk.
   2. Lettuce and fruit.
   3. Eggs, cheese, and enriched bread.
   4. Chicken, spinach, and raisins.

   Answer: 4

   Rationale: Chicken, green leafy vegetables, and dried fruits are all good sources of iron.

   Client Need: Physiological Integrity

   > **Did you remember to choose chicken for great nutritional value?**

44. A client is to be transferred from the intensive care unit to the cardiac step-down unit. The transfer nurse provides pertinent data to the nurse receiving the client. It is vital to include all the following information **except**

   1. The client has a do not resuscitate order.
   2. The client's intravenous bag was hung at 7 a.m. and is running at a KVO (keep vein open) rate.
   3. The client's urinary output was 350 ml today.
   4. The client is married and lives in a one-story home.

   Answer: 4

Rationale: Answers 1, 2, and 3 are pertinent to know for continuity of client care. Knowing that the client is married and the type of dwelling the client lives in does not add to continuity of care.

Client Need: Safe Effective Care Environment

45. Which of the following activities would be *least* helpful in trying to prevent sensory deprivation for a client on bed rest in a private room?

1. Listening to his radio.
2. Reading the newspaper.
3. Keeping the door closed for privacy.
4. Having family members visit.

Answer: 3

Rationale: Clients in private rooms whose doors are closed often experience feelings of isolation and sensory deprivation. Listening to the radio, reading the paper, and talking with visitors does not exhaust the client and helps to decrease sensory deprivation.

> **Did you notice the *emphasized* word? It was meant to help you choose the right answer.**

Client Need: Psychosocial Integrity

46. A 58-year-old woman is brought to the emergency room after being involved in a motor vehicle accident. Shortly after admission, the client's husband arrives. He is distraught and is blaming himself for the accident because he did not drive her himself. What is the nurse's **most appropriate initial** response?

1. Reassure the husband that his wife will be fine.
2. Allow the husband to see his wife immediately.
3. Detail the wife's injuries and plan for treatment.
4. Allow the husband to verbalize his feelings and fears.

Answer: 4

Rationale: Verbalization of feelings and fears is best for the husband. The nurse cannot know the outcome of the client's injuries. The husband is not asking for details at this time and should be calm when he sees his wife.

> Did you notice the key words in the stem to help you find the correct answer?

Client Need: Psychosocial Integrity

---

47. A postterm primigravida woman comes to the antepartum clinic and states she believes she is in labor. The certified nurse midwife examines the client and determines she is in early labor. Which of the following findings **best** indicate true labor?

1. Cervical effacement and dilatation.
2. Fetal descent to 1+ station.
3. Contractions that are painful and occurring every 3 to 4 minutes.
4. The presence of amniotic fluid in the vaginal vault.

Answer: 1

Rationale: The only acceptable indication of true labor is cervical changes. Descent of the fetus, uterine contractions, and rupture of membranes do not indicate true labor.

Client Need: Health Promotion and Maintenance

---

48. Which of the following is considered the highest priority during the first 24 hours postoperatively for the client who has had a thyroidectomy?

1. Patency of airway.
2. Minimal bleeding.
3. Return of the gag reflex.
4. Pain control.

Answer: 1

Rationale: Patency of the airway for the client with surgery of the neck is a priority. Controlling bleeding, return of the gag reflex, and control of pain are important but not the priority.

Client Need: Physiological Integrity

> **Did you remember the ABCs: airway, breathing, and circulation?**

49.   A client receives a wrong medication. The nurse responsible for the medication error should do which of the following *first*?

1. Call the client's physician.
2. Assess the condition of the client.
3. Notify the nursing supervisor.
4. Fill out an incident report.

Answer: 2

Rationale: The priority action for the nurse is to determine if there are any untoward reactions to the medication. The physician and nursing supervisor will eventually have to be called and an incident report will have to be completed, but these are not the priority.

Client Need: Safe Effective Care Environment

50.   A nursery nurse is assigned to a neonate who is 24 hours old. The nurse must perform all of the following actions. Prioritize the following nursing actions in the order the nurse would complete them.

___ Weigh the neonate.
___ Assess the pulse.
___ Assess the respirations.
___ Assess the temperature.
___ Provide cord care.
___ Feed the infant a formula bottle.

Answer: 4, 2, 1, 3, 5, 6

Rationale: Vital signs are completed first. Assessment of respirations is done without disturbing the newborn followed by assessment of the apical pulse. The temperature is taken next. The newborn can be weighed and given cord care next. The infant should be fed last so that sleep will be undisturbed after the feeding.

Client Need: Safe Effective Care Environment

---

51.   A client comes to the clinic after insertion of a permanent pacemaker for postoperative assessment. Which of the following instructions should the nurse include in the client's teaching plan? Select all that apply.

1. Count the heart rate for 1 minute each morning.
2. Count the respiratory rate for 1 minute each morning.
3. Call the clinic if there is redness or swelling at the insertion site.
4. Avoid coming into contact with metal detectors.
5. Avoid microwave ovens.

Answers: 1, 3, and 5

Rationale: A client with a permanent pacemaker should count their heart rate daily and record the information. The nurse should teach the importance of reporting a heart rate that is too slow or too fast. The nurse should also teach the client the signs and symptoms of potential infection at the insertion site. Microwave ovens have been known to disrupt the functioning of the pacemaker. Assessing the respiratory rate is not necessary, and metal detectors will not harm the pacemaker.

Client Need: Physiological Integrity

---

52.   A gravida 1 para 0 client is admitted to the hospital in active labor. Her labor progresses normally, and she delivers a 7 pound 2 ounce healthy baby boy. Two hours after delivery, the nurse assesses that the client has saturated two perineal pads with blood in a 30-minute period. Which action is the **priority** for the nurse to take at this time?

1. Assess the consistency of the client's uterine fundus.
2. Have the client void on the bedpan.
3. Assess the client's vital signs.
4. Notify the delivery physician immediately.

Answer: 1

Rationale: The priority nursing assessment is the consistency of the client's uterine fundus. By assessing the consistency of the client's uterine fundus, the nurse may be able to control the bleeding by massage. If the fundus is not firm, fundal massage may stimulate the fundus to contract, therefore reducing bleeding. The nurse would only have the client void after assessing the fundus. Assessing to see if the fundus is boggy takes priority over the client's vital signs. Calling the physician is appropriate only after assessment of the client.

> Have you been watching for words in the questions that are in **bold**, *italics*, or are <u>underlined</u>? Remember, the purpose of these words is to help you find the correct answer.

Client Need: Health Promotion and Maintenance

53. A client receiving a tap water enema begins to complain of cramping. After a few minutes, he asks the nurse to stop the enema and allow him to go to the bathroom. What would be the nurse's *best* response?

1. Remove the enema and assist the client to the bathroom.
2. Stop the enema briefly and have the client deep breathe.
3. Continue the enema and reassure the client.
4. Stop the enema long enough to give the client pain medication.

Answer: 2

Rationale: If a client complains of cramping during the administration of an enema, the nurse should stop the infusion and have the client deep breathe. Once the cramping is relieved, administration of the enema may continue.

Client Need: Physiological Integrity

54. A newborn nursery nurse is to make rounds. What is the best nursing action to prevent the spread of infection in a newborn nursery?

    1. Hand washing after assessing each baby.
    2. Wearing gloves at all times.
    3. Discarding used pacifiers after each day and replacing them with new ones.
    4. Keeping the bassinets at least 5 feet apart from each other.

    Answer: 1

    Rationale: Hand washing is the number one way of presenting nosocomial infections and spread of infection. Gloves are not always necessary. Pacifiers do not need to be discarded and changed daily. Bassinets do not need to be kept 5 feet apart.

    > Did you remember that hand washing is the priority?

    Client Need: Safe Effective Care Environment

55. A child has just undergone repair of a cleft palate. The surgeon orders restraints. The nurse knows the most appropriate type of restraint for this child is which of the following?

    1. Elbow.
    2. Vest.
    3. Wrist.
    4. Four point.

Answer: 1

Rationale: Elbow restraints are the preferred restraints and effectively prevent the child from placing any fingers in the mouth. Wrist, vest, and four point restraints are too restrictive.

Client Need: Safe Effective Care Environment

---

56.   A client working at a chemical plant was caught in an explosion. He was rescued by his coworkers and presents in the emergency department with third-degree chemical burns over more than 25% of his body. What is the **priority** nursing intervention for this client?

1. Fluid resuscitation.
2. Medicate for pain.
3. Administer tetanus toxoid.
4. Establish and maintain a patent airway.

Answer: 4

Rationale: Establishing an airway is the priority nursing intervention. The client needs fluid resuscitation, pain medication, and a tetanus booster, but these are not the priority.

Ah-ha! Go ahead and stretch and deep breathe.

Client Need: Physiological Integrity

---

57.   A client is diagnosed with fibrocystic breast disease. When teaching the client about dietary changes to help in the treatment of the disease, the nurse should instruct the client to do which of the following?

1. Increase sodium in her diet.
2. Drink only bottled water.
3. Limit her intake of calcium.
4. Decrease her intake of caffeine.

Answer: 4

Rationale: Studies have shown that decreasing caffeine in the diet has been beneficial in the treatment of fibrocystic breast disease in women. It is not advisable to increase sodium and to decrease calcium. Drinking only bottled water is not necessary.

> Did you choose the answer that was generally good for the client?

Client Need: Health Promotion and Maintenance

---

58. A young child is admitted to the pediatric unit and begins to act out. The mother tells the nurse she is afraid the child will not calm down and will be out of control during procedures. The nurse discusses the anticipated care the child will need. Which of the following responses by the parents supports the child's need to be comforted? Select all that apply.

1. A parent stays with the child during procedures.
2. The parents leave the room when the child has an intervention.
3. The parents bring the child's sibling to visit.
4. The parents bring the child's favorite stuffed animal to the hospital.
5. The parents carefully explain all procedures to the child.

Answers: 1, 3, and 4

Rationale: Staying with the child, having a sibling visit, and bringing the child's favorite stuffed animal will soothe the child. The hospitalized child who is alone during painful procedures will feel abandoned. Children at this stage cannot understand detailed explanations about procedures.

Client Need: Psychosocial Integrity

59. A 40-year-old woman has been diagnosed with cancer. She has been advised by her physician to start chemotherapy. The client is concerned about chemotherapy and wants to try nontraditional treatments first. The nurse's **best** response to this client is which of the following?

    1. "Taking nontraditional treatments may place your life in danger."
    2. "Nontraditional treatments are seldom approved by the Food and Drug Administration."
    3. "Nontraditional treatments are seldom used with cancer."
    4. "Tell me more about your concerns about taking chemotherapy."

Answer: 4

Rationale: Asking the client to talk more about her fears and her concerns encourages communication. It is not wise to tell a client they are making a mistake. Telling client's they are mistaken by taking a nontraditional treatment is being judgmental. Stating that nontraditional methods have not been researched with clients with cancer is also judgmental.

Client Need: Safe Effective Care Environment

60. A woman 38 weeks pregnant comes into the prenatal clinic for a contraction stress test. The test results are negative. Which of the following is the nurse's *next* action?

    1. Assess the status of the client's membranes.
    2. Assess the status of the fetus.
    3. Assess if the contractions have ceased.
    4. Assess the client's blood pressure.

Answer: 3

Rationale: A contraction stress test determines the fetus' tolerance to uterine contractions. Therefore it is necessary to assess that the contractions have ceased once the test is completed. Ruptured membranes are seldom associated with a contraction stress test. The status of the fetus and the maternal vital signs are monitored during the contraction stress test.

Client Need: Physiological Integrity

---

61.   The nurse is caring for a child immediately after undergoing a tonsillectomy. The priority assessment for the nurse is to monitor for signs of hemorrhage. This includes which of the following?

   1.   Breathing through the mouth.
   2.   Frequent swallowing.
   3.   The child asking for a drink.
   4.   The child wanting to sleep.

Answer: 2

Rationale: The number one indication of hemorrhage after a tonsillectomy is frequent swallowing. As blood and mucus mix, secretions increase and the client begins to swallow frequently. Breathing through the mouth, complaining of thirst, and wanting to sleep postoperatively are not indications of hemorrhage.

Client Needs: Physiological Integrity

---

62.   The nurse notices that her client receiving a transfusion is having a reaction. The priority nursing intervention includes *all but which* of the following?

   1.   Discontinue the current intravenous site and restart an infusion at a different site.
   2.   Start an intravenous infusion of normal saline to run at 30 ml per hour.
   3.   Assess the client's vital signs every 5 minutes.
   4.   Prepare the blood bag and blood slip to be returned to the blood bank.

Answer: 1

Rationale: It is not advisable to discontinue the intravenous site to restart a new site. The intravenous line should be maintained so that the client can receive the fluids necessary.

Client Need: Physiological Integrity

---

63. One method of calculating a pediatric dose is to divide the child's age by the child's age plus 12. Example: A 4-year-old child would receive the following fraction of the adult dose: $4/(4 + 12) = \frac{4}{16} = \frac{1}{4}$ the adult dose. The result is the fraction of the adult dose safe to give to the child. This method is known as

_____.

Answer: Young's rule

Rationale: Thomas Young is the founder of this formula which is widely used in pediatric settings.

Client Need: Physiological Integrity

---

64. A nurse is caring for a postoperative client. The nurse knows that the most reliable indication of the existence and intensity of the client's acute pain is which of the following?

1. Assessment of the client's vital signs.
2. The client self-reporting of pain.
3. A visual assessment of the client.
4. The severity of the surgical procedure causing the pain.

Ah-ha! Did you remember to take some deep breaths and stretch after answering this question?

Answer: 2

Rationale: The client self-reporting of pain has long been considered the most reliable indicator of the existence of pain and intensity of the pain. It is common practice to have a client rate the level of pain on a scale of 1 to 10, with 10 representing severe pain.

Client Need: Physiological Integrity

65.   A neonate is diagnosed with newborn apnea. Which statement made by the parents reflects an understanding of infant cardiopulmonary resuscitation (CPR)?

    1. "I will use the tips of two fingers to compress the chest."
    2. "I will only blow into the nose."
    3. "I will press the heel of my hand into the sternum."
    4. "Only one of us needs to be CPR certified."

Answer: 1

Rationale: The tips of two fingers are used to compress the chest of an infant. The rescuer should blow into the nose and mouth. The heel of one hand is used for children over the age of 8. It is vital for each parent/caregiver to be CPR certified.

Client Need: Physiological Integrity

---

66.   A 78-year-old woman is admitted to your unit with a fracture of the femur. When assessing the client the nurse suspects a fat embolism. Which of the following assessments will the nurse consider the **earliest** symptom of low arterial blood flow?

    1. Respiratory distress.
    2. Confusion.
    3. Cyanosis.
    4. A temperature of 101.8° F.

Answer: 2

Rationale: Although low arterial blood flow is only one symptom associated with a fat embolism, the earliest indication of this condition is confusion.

> **Did you remember that physiological changes are not considered *early* symptoms?**

Client Need: Physiological Integrity

67. The nurse is completing routine health evaluations on school-aged children. Which of the following alerts the school nurse to the possibility of head lice (pediculosis)?

   1. Patches of baldness.
   2. Blisters on the scalp.
   3. Complaints of scalp itchiness.
   4. Dry patches on the scalp.

Answer: 3

Rationale: The most common indication of head lice in school-aged children is complaints of itchiness and excessive scratching of the scalp.

Client Need: Physiological Integrity

> Ah-ha! Did you remember to stretch and deep breathe after answering this question?

68. A client who is 20 weeks pregnant comes for her prenatal checkup and wants to discuss exercising. She is concerned about the safety of her baby. Which response by the nurse is **most** informative?

   1. "You should not exercise. If you must, do stretches only."
   2. "Exercises you have done routinely can be continued in moderation."
   3. "It is best to do your exercising outdoors."
   4. "You should include a long rest before each new activity."

Answer: 2

Rationale: The client should be informed that participating in her usual activities in moderation is recommended. Stretching activities and bending activities are safe in pregnancy. Pregnant women can exercise indoors or outdoors, and a woman should be told to rest when she feels the need.

Client Need: Health Promotion and Maintenance

69. The nurse is caring for an elderly woman who is underweight and who has been confined to her bed for over a week. Which of the following clinical manifestations best indicates to the nurse that the client may be in the early stages of developing pneumonia?

1. A temperature of greater than 101°F and complaints of chills.
2. A productive cough.
3. Confusion.
4. Complaints of chest pain.

> **Did you remember that one of the earliest signs of decreased oxygen saturation is confusion?**

Answer: 3

Rationale: One of the earliest indications of decreased arterial oxygen saturation is confusion.

Client Need: Physiological Integrity

70. The nurse on the pediatric unit is caring for a child who is receiving a unit of packed red blood cells. Within minutes, the child becomes restless and has difficulty breathing. The nurse takes immediate action to ensure the safety and well-being of the child. Arrange the following numbered nursing actions from highest to lowest priority.

1. Call the pediatrician.
2. Prepare to perform CPR.
3. Place the child in an oxygen tent.
4. Stop the blood and administer normal saline.
5. Assess the child's vital signs.

Answer: 4, 3, 5, 1, 2

Rationale: The nurse's immediate response is to stop administering the blood and begin administering normal saline. The nurse would then give the child oxygen and then assess the child vital signs. Next, the pediatrician is notified. Preparing to perform CPR comes last.

Client Need: Safe Effective Care Environment

71. A diabetic client's morning blood glucose concentration was inaccurately documented as 210 instead of 120 on the client's chart. The nurse did not notice the error until after the client had eaten breakfast. The nurse had already administered a sliding scale dose of insulin for a blood glucose level of 210. What is the nurse's *next priority* action?

1. Call the house physician.
2. Assess the client for signs of hypoglycemia.
3. Complete an incident report.
4. Notify the nursing supervisor.

Answer: 2

Rationale: It is vital that the client be assessed for signs of hypoglycemia. Notifying the doctor, completing an incident report, and calling the nursing supervisor can be done later.

> Did you remember that nurses Assess Before Caring?

Client Need: Physiological Integrity

72. A 60-year-old woman is admitted to the hospital with a diagnosis of breast cancer. She is scheduled to have a modified radical mastectomy. The client appears anxious and is asking many questions. The nurse's **best** response is to do which of the following?

1. Answer as many of the client's questions as possible.
2. Avoid discussing the client's questions until she is calm.
3. Ask the client to direct her questions to the surgeon.
4. Delay answering the client's questions until preoperative medication is administered.

Answer: 1

Rationale: An important part of preoperative teaching is to answer as many questions as the client has to the nurse's best ability. Avoiding answering her questions and referring her to the surgeon is not accepting responsibility for the client's welfare. After giving preoperative medication, the client's ability to understand will diminish.

Client Need: Psychosocial Integrity

---

73.   A client in a nursing home is receiving a nasogastric tube feeding. Which of the following nursing actions is the **priority** for the nurse to complete before administering the tube feeding?

1. Warm the feeding solution in a microwave oven.
2. Place the client in a low Fowler's position.
3. Aspirate residual gastric contents and discard.
4. Verify the correct positioning of the feeding tube.

Answer: 4

Rationale: The priority nursing assessment to be completed before administering any feeding is to verify the position of the tube. The solutions are not warmed in a microwave oven. The client's position should be semi- to high Fowler's. The gastric residual is not discarded.

> Did you remember that safety is the priority for clients?

Client Need: Physiological Integrity

---

74.   A postoperative client returns to the unit from the postanesthesia care unit. Which of the following is the nurse's **priority** assessment?

1. The intravenous fluid and intravenous site.
2. The level of the client's pain.
3. The surgical dressing.
4. The patency of the client's nasogastric tube.

Answer: 3

Rationale: The priority is to assess the surgical dressing for bleeding and drainage.

Client Need: Physiological Integrity

> Did you remember your ABCs: airway, breathing, and circulation?

75. An infant returns to the pediatric unit after surgical correction of a tracheal-esophageal fistula. The **priority** nursing diagnosis for this client is which of the following?

1. Risk for infection.
2. Acute postoperative pain.
3. Risk of constipation.
4. Impaired physical mobility.

Answer: 1

Rationale: The risk for infection is a priority diagnosis for the nurse to make. Medicating the infant for pain, observing for signs of constipation, and being aware of the infant's decreased mobility are important but not the priority.

Client Need: Physiological Integrity

> Did you remember that in the absence of airway, breathing, and circulation, infection is often the next priority?

76. The nurse's neighbor comes over to say that she just burned her arm on the stove. The nurse should advise the neighbor to do which of the following *first*?

1. Apply ice to the burn.
2. Apply antibacterial ointment to the burn.
3. Pour cool water over the burn.
4. Wrap the burn in a clean cloth.

Answer: 3

Rationale: It is always advisable to stop the burning process by using cool clean water. Seldom are extreme temperatures, such as ice, advisable. Oils can continue to heat up and cause continuation of the burning process.

Client Need: Physiological Integrity

> Did you remember that nurses do not use hot or cold applications but rather cool or warm?

77. The nurse enters a client's room to administer the 8 a.m. medications and notices that the client is in an awkward position in bed and has not eaten breakfast. What is the nurse's *priority* action?

1. Ask the client to state his name.
2. Feed the client his breakfast.
3. Correct the client's position in bed.
4. Administer the client's medications.

Answer: 3

Rationale: Correcting the client's position is the priority to increase the client's level of comfort and maintain the client's airway.

Client Need: Physiological Integrity

78. An infant is admitted to the hospital with infectious meningitis. On assessment, the nurse notices the infant cries when he flexes and then extends his legs. The nurse correctly documents this as _____.

Answer: Kernig's sign

Rationale: Kernig's sign is only one of several indicators of meningitis.

Client Need: Physiological Integrity

79.   The nurse is assessing a client who delivered vaginally 3 hours earlier and notes the following: The fundus is displaced to the right of midline, is firm, and is two finger breaths above the umbilicus. Based on these findings which action is *most* appropriate for the nurse to take initially?

1. Massage the uterine fundus.
2. Notify the physician.
3. Have the client void.
4. Document the assessments in the client's chart.

Answer: 3

Rationale: A full bladder displaces the uterine fundus and elevates it above the level of the umbilicus. Having the client void allows the uterus to settle back to midline below the umbilicus. There is no reason to massage the fundus because the nurse found it to be firm. There is no reason to notify the physician. Correction of the displaced uterus is the nurse's priority. Documenting information can be done after the finding has been corrected.

Client Need: Health Promotion and Maintenance

80.   A 26-year-old man is diagnosed with gout. He comes to the health care clinic and the physician orders allopurinol (Zyloprim). Which statement, if made by the client, indicates to the nurse that the client understands the proper way to take this medication?

1. "If I get a rash that is itchy, I will take my usual antihistamine."
2. "I need to drink at least 3000 ml a day while taking allopurinol."
3. "I should take the medicine on an empty stomach."
4. "If I develop any hives or my lips swell, I should put an ice pack on them."

Answer: 2

Rationale: Clients who take allopurinol (Zyloprim) are encouraged to drink at least 3000 ml each day. The drug should be given with food or milk or immediately after a meal. If the client develops itchy eyes, hives, a

rash, or swelling of the tongue, the physician should be contacted immediately because this may indicate an allergic reaction.

Client Need: Health Promotion and Maintenance

81. A toddler is diagnosed with strep throat. The pediatrician orders amoxicillin
or Augmentin 300 mg orally four times a day. The pharmacist sends a bottle
labeled 250 mg per 5 ml. How many milliliters should the nurse administer
for each dose?

_____

Answer: 6

Rationale: The pediatrician has ordered 300 mg divided by 250 mg and
multiplied by 5 ml. The correct amount is 6 ml.

Client Need: Physiological Integrity

82. A visiting nurse goes to the home of a client who has been diagnosed with
chronic obstructive pulmonary disease (COPD). The client is on home oxygen
at 2 l per minute via nasal cannula. The client tells the nurse she has been experiencing difficulty breathing or dyspnea. Which nursing action is the **priority**
for the visiting nurse at this time?

1. Increase the client's oxygen to 3 l per minute.
2. Perform a respiratory assessment.
3. Call 911 and have the client brought to the emergency department.
4. Contact the client's physician.

Answer: 2

Rationale: Completing a respiratory assessment and collecting subjective and objective information regarding the client's respiratory status is the nurse's priority inter-

> **Did you remember
> that nurses Assess
> Before Caring?**

vention. Once the nurse completes the assessment, the physician can be called. Dialing 911 would be premature at this time. The flow of oxygen is not increased for clients with COPD because of carbon dioxide retention.

Client Need: Physiological Integrity

83. A 1-day postpartum client requests a warm sitz bath. The nurse is to assess how the client is tolerating the procedure. What is the nurse's *priority* assessment?

1. Ask the client if she feels nauseous.
2. Assess the client's pulse and skin color.
3. Monitor the client's oral temperature and respiratory rate.
4. Assess if the client's pain level is reduced.

Answer: 2

Rationale: A warm sitz bath causes vasodilation; therefore the nurse should monitor the client's pulse rate and skin color. Answers 1 and 3 are not associated with vasodilation. Asking the client if her symptoms are relieved tells the nurse if the treatment is effective and would not indicate how well the client is tolerating the sitz bath.

> Remember, all parts of an answer must be correct in order to choose that answer.

Client Need: Safe Effective Care Environment

84. A postoperative abdominal surgery client is on bed rest. The client calls the nurse and states he needs to urinate and asks for the bedside commode. The nurse is aware the nurse from the previous shift allowed the client to get out of bed and use the commode. The nurse assists the client to the commode, and, consequently, the client sustains an injury to the surgical incision. The nurse could be liable for his or her action according to the definition of which of the following?

1. Tort.
2. Misdemeanor.
3. Statutory law.
4. Common law.

Answer: 1

Rationale: A tort is defined as a wrongful act, done intentionally or unintentionally against a person or a person's property. The nurse's actions in this situation are consistent with the definition of a tort. A misdemeanor is an offense under criminal law.

Client Need: Physiological Integrity

85. A mother of a newborn diagnosed with colic is requesting information about what to do when the newborn is crying. The nurse correctly suggests which of the following? Select all that apply.

1. Burp the infant frequently with each feeding.
2. Bring the infant to the emergency room for evaluation when there is evidence of colic pain.
3. Talking quietly to the infant and rocking often help to soothe a crying baby.
4. Feed the infant small amounts of formula more frequently.
5. Ignore this behavior because it will diminish with time.

Answers: 1, 3, and 4

Rationale: The infant does not require an emergency room visit. Colic will not diminish with time, and ignoring the behavior is neglectful. Frequent burping, rocking movements, and smaller feedings are usually helpful for the infant with colic.

Client Need: Physiological Integrity

86. A client comes to the health care clinic after being diagnosed with peptic ulcer disease. The client is placed on propantheline (Pro-Banthine). The nurse instructs the client on the proper use of the medication by instructing the client to do which of the following?

1. Take the Pro-Banthine with an antacid.
2. Take the medication ½ hour before meals.
3. Take the medication with food or milk.
4. Take the medication after meals.

Answer: 2

Rationale: Pro-Banthine is a medication that decreases gastrointestinal secretions. It is typically administered ½ hour before meals. Answers 1, 3, and 4 are incorrect.

Client Need: Health Promotion and Maintenance

87. A client on your unit is receiving total parenteral nutrition (TPN). You perform a scheduled finger stick on the client and assess the client's serum glucose level at 350 mg/dl. What would be your **initial** nursing intervention?

1. Discontinue the TPN and start infusing D_5W.
2. Decrease the flow rate of the TPN to a KVO (keep vein open) rate.
3. Increase the flow rate of the TPN to 150 ml per hour.
4. Contact the client's physician.

Answer: 4

Rationale: Hyperglycemia is a complication often associated with client's receiving TPN. A glucose level of 350 mg/dl must be reported to the client's physician immediately. Answers 1, 2, and 3 require a physician's order.

Client Need: Physiological Integrity

88.   A newly delivered mother is holding her newborn infant and notices that the umbilical cord has been dyed. The mother questions the nurse as to why this has been done. The nurse explains the purpose of using triple dye on the umbilical cord to the mother by stating which of the following?

    1.   "Triple dye is used because it decreases bacterial growth and helps the cord to dry."
    2.   "Triple dye is applied because it helps the cord drop off in less than 5 days."
    3.   "If we did not use triple dye on the cord the baby might hemorrhage."
    4.   "Triple dye is applied to the cord because it helps us see the blood vessels better."

Answer: 1

Rationale: The umbilical cord begins to dry at the time of birth. Triple dye helps to decrease bacterial growth and aids in the drying of the cord, although some hospitals have discontinued its use. Answers 2, 3, and 4 are incorrect.

Client Need: Physiological Integrity

89.   A 52-year-old man is admitted to the cardiac care unit with a diagnosis of premature ventricular contractions. The client has an order to be out of bed in a chair twice a day. When the client is sitting in the chair, he suddenly begins to complain of feeling lightheaded. The nurse takes the client's apical pulse and is likely to detect which of the following?

    1.   A regular apical pulse.
    2.   An irregular apical pulse.
    3.   Tachycardia.
    4.   Bradycardia.

Answer: 2

Rationale: The most accurate means to assess a client's heart rate and rhythm is to auscultate the client's apical pulse. When a client is experiencing premature ventricular contractions, the apical pulse rate will be irregular and the client may complain of lightheadedness.

Client Need: Physiological Integrity

90. A client comes to the outpatient clinic and is scheduled to have a barium swallow the next day. The nurse provides the client with preprocedure instructions. Which statement, if made by the client, indicates to the nurse that teaching was successful?

1. "I should take all my oral medications before I come in the morning."
2. "I will chart my bowel movements for the past week and bring it with me tomorrow."
3. "I will remove my metal jewelry before coming tomorrow morning."
4. "I will make sure I eat a good breakfast tomorrow because I will probably be here for a long time."

Answer: 3

Rationale: A barium swallow is an x-ray that highlights abnormalities of the gastrointestinal tract. The client is asked to remove all metal jewelry that may interfere with the films. The client will be NPO the morning of the test and should not take anything orally. The client will be taught to watch for constipation postprocedure.

Did you use "good" and "bad" to answer this question?

Client Need: Physiological Integrity

91. A physician orders medications for a client newly admitted to your unit. On review of the physician's orders, you notice the dose is three times normal. You call the physician's office and are told he will not be available for several days. What is your **next priority** nursing intervention?

   1. Contact the pharmacy and confirm the dosage is safe to administer.
   2. Withhold the medication until the ordering physician can be reached.
   3. Contact the answering service and speak with the covering on-call physician.
   4. Document your concerns and administer the medication as ordered.

Answer: 3

Rationale: When a nurse believes there has been an error with a physician's order, it is the nurse's responsibility to clarify the order before carrying it out. The nurse may confirm the dose with the pharmacy but is not authorized to adjust the dosage. It is not appropriate to wait a length of time to speak to a physician. It is also inappropriate to document your concerns and administer the medication in this situation.

Client Need: Safe Effective Care Environment

92. A client newly diagnosed with gastroesophageal reflux disease (GERD) has just been discharged from the hospital. During discharge teaching the nurse clarifies the physician's orders for at-home care. Which comment, if made by the client, indicates to the nurse that teaching has been effective?

   1. "I will lay on my left side to sleep at night."
   2. "I will lay on my right side to sleep at night."
   3. "I will sleep on my back with my head on a pillow."
   4. "I will sleep on my stomach with my head flat."

Answer: 1

Rationale: Clients diagnosed with gastroesophageal reflux should be instructed to sleep on their left side with the head slightly elevated. This position helps to relieve one of the most common complaints associated with GERD, which is heartburn.

Client Need: Physiological Integrity

93. The nurse knows that clients who undergo transurethral resection of the prostate frequently experience postoperative pain caused by what common physiological response to the surgery?

_____

Answer: Bladder spasms

Rationale: Bladder spasms are the most common cause of postoperative pain in clients who have undergone transurethral resection of the prostate.

Client Need: Physiological Integrity

94. The nursing instructor is teaching a class of students about clients who suffer with uncontrolled vomiting and diarrhea. The instructor correctly points out that the priority assessments for clients with this condition are which of the following? Select all that apply.

1. Poor skin turgor.
2. Bradycardia.
3. Hypotension.
4. Sunken eyes.
5. Lethargy.

Answers: 1, 3, 4, and 5

Rationale: Clients with uncontrolled vomiting and diarrhea will most like become dehydrated. Weight loss, lethargy, sunken eyes, poor skin turgor, tachycardia, and hypotension are classic indicators of dehydration.

Client Need: Physiological Integrity

95. A client is admitted to your unit and is ordered to be on intake and output. The client consumes the following fluids the morning of your shift:

1 cup of coffee

4 ounces of orange juice

3 ounces of water

1 cup of jello

1 cup of tea

5 ounces of broth

3 ounces of water

When totaling the client's fluid intake for your shift, how many milliliters would you record on the client's intake and output record?

Answer: 1170

Rationale: 1 cup is the equivalent of 8 ounces. 1 ounce is the equivalent of 30 ml. When adding the fluids together, the total is 1170 ml.

Did you remember *not* to label your answer? The label was included in the stem of the question.

Client Need: Physiological Integrity

96. The nurse is caring for her newly delivered client on the postpartum unit. Which signs and symptoms indicate to the nurse the presence of a possible abnormality in the postpartum recovering client?

1. The client experienced chills shortly after delivery.
2. The client's pulse rate is 60.
3. The client's urinary output is 3000 ml.
4. The client's oral temperature is 101°F.

Answer: 4

Rationale: An oral body temperature greater than 100.4°F in the postpartum period indicates the possibility of a postpartum infection. Chills shortly after delivery is considered normal, and a heart rate of 60 beats per minute the day after delivery is not abnormal. Postpartum clients diurese to rid the body of excess fluids retained in pregnancy. Therefore, a urinary output of up to 3000 ml per day is normal following the delivery of a baby.

Client Need: Safe Effective Care Environment

97. A 36-year-old woman has undergone a left radical mastectomy for invasive cancer. The nurse correctly interprets that the client is having difficulty adjusting to the loss of her breast if which of the following behaviors is observed?

1. The client refuses to look at the dressing or surgical incision.
2. The client is asking for pain medication every 3 hours.
3. The client is asking questions about the information on her postoperative care pamphlet.
4. The client is performing arm exercises only once a shift.

Answer: 1

Rationale: Clients who refuse to look at the surgical incision or surgical dressing are having difficulty adjusting to the loss of a body part or with body disfigurement. This indicates the client is not yet ready to acknowledge the results of the surgery. Asking for pain medication, performing arm exercises, and wanting postoperative care information are positive signs indicating adjustments to the postoperative period.

Did you notice the word "only" in answer 4?

Client Need: Psychosocial Integrity

98. The nurse in the neonatal intensive care unit is informed that a newborn with an Apgar score of 2 and 5 will be brought to the unit. The nurse prepares for the arrival of the newborn by completing all the following interventions. Prioritize the interventions in the order the nurse would complete them.

___ Turn on the digital newborn scale.
___ Turn on the apnea and cardiac/respiratory monitor.
___ Set up an intravenous line of D_5W.
___ Prepare a newborn Ambu resuscitation bag with oxygen.
___ Turn on the radiant warmer control to a temperature of 97.6°F.

Answer: 5, 2, 3, 1, 4

Rationale: The nurse first prepares to resuscitate the infant (Airway) and next sets up the apnea and cardiac/respiratory monitor (Breathing). Next, the nurse sets up an intravenous line of D_5W (Circulation), followed by turning on the radiant warmer. The last step the nurse completes is turning on the digital scale.

> Did you remember Airway, Breathing, and Circulation?

Client Need: Physiological Integrity

99. Your client has undergone a transurethral prostatectomy. During discharge teaching, the nurse informs the client that he should expect which of the following variations in normal urine color?

1. Pale pink.
2. Bright yellow.
3. Bright red.
4. Dark amber.

Answer: 1

Rationale: The postoperative client who is going home should be told to expect urine that is pale pink. If the client's urine turns red or bright red, he should be instructed to notify his physician immediately.

Client Need: Physiological Integrity

---

100.   A 9-year-old boy is newly diagnosed with diabetes and tells the nurse he is anxious to return to school and participate in social events. The mother of the young boy tells the nurse she is hesitant to send him to school and does not want him taking part in any physical activities. What is the nurse's *most* appropriate response to the mother?

1.   "Tell me more about how you are feeling."
2.   "It is okay for you to have him home-schooled using tutors."
3.   "I agree. His well-being is the most important."
4.   "You sound overprotective. Let's talk about this some more."

Answer: 1

Rationale: Asking the mother to talk more about her feelings encourages communication. You should never tell a mother whether you agree or disagree. Telling a mother she is overprotective will not foster communication and trust.

Client Need: Psychosocial Integrity

---

101.   A physician orders 2 g of the medication to be given to a client in the next 24 hours in eight divided doses. The nurse knows to administer how much medication for each of the eight doses?

_____

Answer: 250 mg

Did you remember to label your answer? It was not included in the question.

Rationale: First, convert the 2 g to mg, which equates to 2000 mg. Next, simply divide the 2000 mg by 8. The answer is 250 mg.

Ah-ha! Did you remember to stretch and deep breathe? Refresh yourself.

Client Need: Physiological Integrity

---

102. A client is to receive a unit of packed red blood cells. The nurse knows that in setting up the intravenous solution, the solution of choice is

1. Ringer's lactate.
2. Normal saline.
3. Dextrose 5% in water.
4. Dextrose 5% in ½ normal saline.

Answer: 2

Rationale: Normal saline is the only fluid that may be administered with blood products such as packed red blood cells because it does not cause clotting of the blood components. Answers 1, 3, and 4 cause clotting of the blood components.

Client Need: Safe Effective Care Environment

---

103. A newly delivered mother who is gravida 5 para 5 asks the nurse about information concerning oral contraceptives. Which statement made by the mother indicates to the nurse that she has understood the teaching about oral contraceptives?

1. "Oral contraceptives work best with women whose menstrual cycles are regular."
2. "Oral contraceptives are more effective in women who are younger."
3. "Oral contraceptives are very effective when taken as the doctor prescribes."
4. "Oral contraceptives work best when used with other birth control devices such as spermicides and diaphragms."

Answer: 3

Rationale: Oral contraceptives are effective approximately 95% to 99% of the time when taken as directed by the physician. Answers 1, 2, and 4 are not relevant to oral contraceptives.

Client Need: Health Promotion and Maintenance

---

104. A cardiac client is to receive Lasix (furosemide) 40 mg by mouth. The nurse notes that the client has not been receiving supplemental electrolytes. Which laboratory value is a *priority* for the nurse to assess before administering the Lasix?

_____

Answer: Potassium

Rationale: Lasix is a loop diuretic and therefore promotes excretion of potassium. The nurse should monitor the client's serum potassium level before administering the Lasix to prevent hypokalemia.

Client Need: Physiological Integrity

---

105. A female client is admitted to the emergency room after being attacked by a stranger. She told police she was robbed and raped at knifepoint. The client appears calm and is sitting quietly in the exam room. The nurse correctly identifies her behavior as the protective defense mechanism known as _____.

Answer: Denial

Rationale: Denial is a protective defense mechanism that assists the client in consciously refusing to acknowledge unspeakable thoughts and images. It is a common response for sexually abused victims.

Client Need: Psychosocial Integrity

106. The pediatric nurse correctly identifies which muscle as the preferred site for intramuscular injections in infants under 1 year of age?

_____

Answer: Vastus lateralis

Rationale: The vastus lateralis is preferred in infants under the age of 1 year because of the limited amount of nerve endings and major blood vessels. Other sites may be used once the child is walking.

Client Need: Physiological Integrity

107. A client newly diagnosed with gastroesophageal disease (GERD) has just been discharged from the hospital. During discharge teaching the client asks the nurse which foods he should avoid eating. The nurse instructs the client to avoid certain foods. Which foods, if chosen by the client for lunch, indicate to the nurse that further teaching is not necessary? Select all that apply.

1. Nonfat milk.
2. Chocolate.
3. Coffee.
4. Fried eggs.
5. Dry whole wheat toast.

Answers: 1 and 5

Rationale: Foods that are low in fat increase lower esophageal sphincter pressure and lessen the symptoms of GERD. Foods such as chocolate, coffee, fatty foods, and alcoholic beverages decrease lower esophageal sphincter pressure and amplify the symptoms of GERD.

Client Need: Physiological Integrity

108.   A woman 30 weeks gestation is admitted to the maternity unit in preterm labor. The obstetrician orders betamethasone (Celestone) to be administered stat to the mother. The mother asks the nurse about the purpose of the medication. The nurse correctly tells the mother the medication is used for which of the following reasons?

    1. To stop preterm labor contractions.
    2. To stop cervical dilation.
    3. To boost fetal lung maturity.
    4. To increase the fetal heart.

Answer: 3

Rationale: Betamethasone (Celestone) is a corticosteroid that boosts fetal lung maturity. Answers 1, 2, and 4 are incorrect.

Did step 5 help you here?

Client Need: Physiological Integrity

109.   A physician orders a client to have an intravenous line started with 500 ml of D_5W with 40 mEq of KCl to infuse at 10 mEq per hour. The drop factor on the tubing is 10. The nurse knows to correctly run the intravenous line at what rate?

_____

Answer: 21 gtts/min

Rationale: The nurse first needs to know how many milliliters is takes to deliver 10 mEq of KCl. A ratio and proportion is used to show that 40 mEq is to 500 ml as 10 mEq is to X ml. The result is 125 ml. The next step is to simply plug the correct numbers into the IV formula, such as 125 ml is divided by 60 minutes (time) and multiplied by 10 (drop factor). The answer is 21 gtts/min.

Did you remember to label your answer? The label was *not* included in the stem of the question.

Client Need: Physiological Integrity

110.   A 46-year-old man is admitted with complaints of abdominal distention. A nasogastric tube is inserted and connected to low gastric suction. Shortly after admission, the client begins to complain of discomfort and a feeling of bloating. Which of the following assessments is the *priority* for the nurse to make?

1. Notify the client's physician.
2. Irrigate the nasogastric tube with 100 ml of sterile water.
3. Check to see if the suction equipment is working.
4. Remove and reinsert the nasogastric tube.

Answer: 3

Rationale: Assessing to see if the suction equipment is in working order is the nurse's first action. Answers 1, 2, and 4 are interventions, not assessments.

> Did you remember the ABCs: nurses Assess Before Caring?